Dedication

This book was made possible because of four people: many thanks to RGS and MRS for encouragement and time; much appreciation to BRG for insight and patience; volumes of gratitude to GRG for emphasizing accountability; and love to all.

JGS

Forward

This book is for anyone who, like me, has fibromyalgia. In addition, this book is appropriate for anyone who cares for, is friends with, or is related to someone with fibromyalgia. Finally, this book is appropriate for anyone who is not sure about whether he or she has fibromyalgia but would like to do some research before going forward to seek a diagnosis.

If you support someone who has fibromyalgia, I hope that you gain a greater understanding of this condition and learn what you might do for the one you support.

If you have fibromyalgia, I trust that by sharing with you how fibromyalgia has affected me, including what science and medicine have to offer us, that you too can live fully with fibromyalgia. My ultimate wish for you is that this information informs you in areas where you require more information, clarifies what is confusing to you, and gives you the hope that fibromyalgia can not only be managed, but also it can be controlled so that you can have an excellent quality of life.

Best wishes,

JG Schnellmann

TABLE OF CONTENTS

Chapter 1— Introduction to Fibromyalgia

What is Fibromyalgia?

Fibromyalgia is a real, persistent condition of pain felt throughout the body.[1, 2] In fact, such pain is the hallmark of fibromyalgia, and this pain can present itself as a burning, stinging, or heavy sensation in the major muscles of the upper body such as the shoulders, neck, and upper back, and of the lower body, including the lower back and legs. For many people with fibromyalgia, such pain is not usually relieved by traditional, over-the-counter pain medicines, and sleep does not seem to reverse the fatigue that is commonly associated with the pain. Increasing the complexity of fibromyalgia, pain and fatigue are often, but not always, accompanied by other bothersome symptoms such as stiffness, swelling of the hands and feet, gastric complaints, headaches, and cold intolerance.

Because many people may not be aware of the breadth of fibromyalgia symptoms, a list of questions related to fibromyalgia is presented below. These questions cover the most common symptoms reported in people with fibromyalgia.

What Does Fibromyalgia Feel Like?

❖ Do you have general and persistent pain throughout your whole body or in your legs, arms, and back muscles that is not the result of an injury?

❖ Is the pain you experience a burning or stinging sensation resembling muscle fatigue from overuse?

❖ Do your limbs often feel heavy and "spent" after little activity?

❖ Do you often feel that simple tasks, such as rising from a chair or pushing a shopping cart, take enormous energy?

❖ Does the pain you have worsen or improve randomly?

❖ Have you had this pain for a long time, with no memorable event that seemed to trigger it?

❖ Along with this muscular pain, are you constantly tired, as if you have not had sleep for days?

❖ Are you mentally foggy, and do you have trouble remembering small things?

❖ When you wake up in the morning, are you just as tired as when you went to bed?

❖ Do your joints feel stiff after rising in the morning?

❖ Do you get up many times during the night to urinate?

❖ Do your hands and feet swell occasionally?

❖ Do you have an irritated stomach sometimes?

❖ Can cold weather make your fingers and toes turn white and numb or tingly?

❖ Are you plagued by migraine headaches?

❖ Finally, when you describe this constant pain and exhaustion to other people, do they look at you as if you have lost your mind?

If many or all of these symptoms apply to you, you may have fibromyalgia—a unique medical condition of constant muscular pain usually accompanied by multiple related symptoms such as headache, mental fogginess, stiffness, frequent urination, upset stomach, and cold intolerance.

How is Fibromyalgia Diagnosed?

Frequently, people who experience chronic and persistent pain in their body accompanied by overall stiffness, swelling in their hands and feet, and relentless fatigue will see a physician about these symptoms, seeking relief and information about why these symptoms are occurring. Physicians who are knowledgeable about fibromyalgia can analyze these symptoms using a set of clinically tested and medically established criteria for the unique disorder of fibromyalgia, and they can differentiate these symptoms from other types of fatigue and pain disorders.

Presently, criteria for fibromyalgia are greatly dependent on complaints of muscular discomfort/pain that has been ongoing for more than three months.[1] To assess the severity of this chronic pain aspect of fibromyalgia, a physician can evaluate the presence of *tender points* which are areas on the body that are painful to the patient when a precise amount of pressure is directly applied to that area—specifically 9 pounds of pressure. After applying the prescribed amount of pressure to the areas depicted in **Figure 1**, the physician asks the patient if there is pain. A positive response from the patient—for example, a statement such as "yes, that causes pain", wincing, jumping, or an exclamation of pain—confirms a tender point.

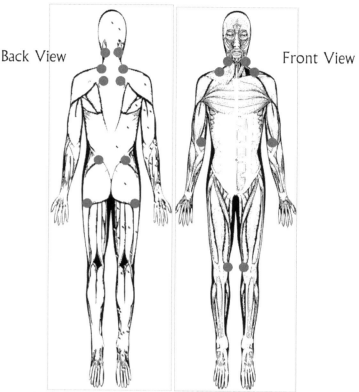

Back View   Front View

● Gray circle denotes location of tender point
Figure 1. Muscles affected in fibromyalgia. Confirmation of 11 of the 18 common tender points is considered diagnostic for fibromyalgia.

A person who reports having pain at 11 of the 18 tender points depicted in **Figure** 1 is considered to have fibromyalgia, and the conclusion of such a diagnosis is strengthened when the patient reports additional symptoms that are commonly associated with fibromyalgia such as unrefreshing sleep, tiredness, and swelling in the hands and feet.[1, 3] However, it should be noted that a diagnosis of fibromyalgia can be made simply by the confirmation of tender points, even when the other symptoms such as fatigue, stiffness, headache, etc, are not present.[4-6] Alternately, many people who do not experience discrete tender points are diagnosed with fibromyalgia.[2] Also, sites of tenderness depicted in **Figure** 1 are considered to be representative—each gray dot in the

Figure does not necessarily indicate an *actual area*, but it suggests a general area. Thus, a person can experience pain *near* or *around* the sites depicted in **Figure 1**, and this will confirm the presence of a tender point.

Of course, for many people, having sufficient pressure applied to some areas of the body can produce pain most of the time, and this idea may be confusing when considering that the presence of painful tender points is a confirmation of fibromyalgia. Thus, the pressure applied in the tender point test is standardized so that physicians will use the same amount of pressure for all patients. To understand how much pressure is applied during the clinical tender point assessment, firmly press your thumb or index finger on a table until the nail bed turns white. This action mimics the approximate pressure applied in the clinical tender point test.

You may notice that **Figure 1** is not labeled with the complicated scientific names of muscles. Rather, **Figure 1** simply depicts areas that you or your physician can target when diagnosing and evaluating your pain. Perhaps the figure will give you a better idea of why your pain seems to be "all over" your body: tender points are distributed so broadly across the body that they can *literally* cause you to interpret your pain as being *everywhere*. So, you are not imagining that you are hurting all over; you really are!

Now that we have addressed the complaints that arise from the profound—and seemingly unexplained—muscular pain of fibromyalgia, we will discuss the other troubling symptoms of fibromyalgia such as stiffness, fatigue, swelling, frequent urination, mental fogginess and forgetfulness, occasional numbness in the fingers and toes, upset stomach or irritable bowels, and headaches.

Signs and Symptoms of Fibromyalgia

The additional symptoms described below are so commonly tied to fibromyalgia that they are often considered part of the fibromyalgia spectrum.[6, 7] Of course, each of these symptoms, by itself, may indicate a unique illness that is unrelated to fibromyalgia. Thus, according to current clinical guidelines, these symptoms *alone* are not sufficient to render a firm verdict of fibromyalgia, but when the symptoms are all analyzed collectively, they are very compelling evidence of fibromyalgia.[8]

❖ Fatigue and Unrefreshing Sleep

Fatigue and non-restorative sleep are hallmarks of fibromyalgia,[9, 10] but they are difficult to tease apart: which one causes the other? It is obvious that lack of restorative sleep would contribute to being tired during the day, and a continuous pattern of poor sleep could eventually manifest in other ways such as headaches, gastric distress, joint pain, etc. Knowledge of how sleep affects fibromyalgia can be gleaned from understanding what normal sleep patterns look like and how the sleep of people with fibromyalgia differs from these normal patterns.

First, sleep is more than lying down and counting sheep. Sleep actually has 4 recognized stages. Stage 1 is marked by a drowsiness in which the brain begins to alter its pattern of processing information. During Stage 1 sleep, people may twitch or jerk as muscles relax and consciousness fades. The longest phase of sleep is Stage 2 (called true sleep) and in this stage, people are unaware of their environment, and muscles are quiet and still. The deepest stage of sleep, Stage 3, is thought to be a transitional stage, and in this phase, sleepwalking, bedwetting in children, and talking in one's sleep are more likely to occur. As Stage 3 progresses to Stage 4, sleep deepens again. Over the night, your sleep cycles among the 4 stages, combined with dream stages, called rapid eye movement (REM) sleep. In REM sleep, we dream, process emotions, relieve stress, and refresh our brain.

Science has shown that people with fibromyalgia have disrupted Stage 2 sleep, along with more wakefulness, longer sleep latency (time to fall asleep), and frequent sleep fragmentation (episodes of waking during sleep).[11-13] Whether a lack of sleep intensifies the symptoms of fibromyalgia or whether fibromyalgia reduces quality of sleep is under investigation. In a study including a small sample of healthy men, sleep deprivation induced *hyperalgesia*, which means that sleep deprivation increased the men's perception of and response to pain.[14-16] Another study including men with sleep apnea—a condition of interrupted breathing that triggers sudden wakefulness—suggests that lack of sleep does *not* contribute to increased pain sensitivity in some individuals, a finding that directly contrasts with the previous study. Yet, men in this sleep apnea study did report increased fatigue.[17] Certainly, more studies to investigate these links are warranted, and these studies should include women. Thus, interrupted sleep may not increase sensitivity to pain, but it may produce fatigue. A less documented phenomena—and perhaps a more unusual idea—is how *fatigue* can disrupt *sleep.*

Fatigue can disturb sleep by not allowing an individual to become sufficiently tired to fall asleep and stay asleep. The daytime is usually a time of activity and motion, and fatigue during the day can prevent a person from exerting physical effort during activities of daily living such as gardening, retrieving the mail, getting the newspaper, shopping, walking, or visiting friends. Also, fatigue can be severe enough to make daily exercise very unpalatable.[18] Many people with fibromyalgia claim to be too tired to exercise, and this lack of movement or purposeful exercise may keep the body from feeling tired enough to rest at night— after all, the body thinks that it has "rested" all day. Thus, when night comes, the body does not truly sense a shift in rhythm.

Interestingly, in studies of the circadian rhythm, which is the body's internal night and day clock, no differences were found between normal women and women with fibromyalgia.[19] Thus, this internal body clock is likely not the culprit of disturbed sleep, but other factors such as lack of exercise or constant pain may be the cause of sleep disruptions.

Pain can disrupt sleep and contribute to daytime fatigue.[20] People with arthritis complain of poor sleep quality because their pain keeps them awake.[14, 21] Pain associated with fibromyalgia can make for restless sleep as one rolls over on painful muscles, awakening in the night.[14] Also, people with fibromyalgia find difficulty in getting comfortable enough to sleep. For example, the positions that relieve pain in the legs and back may not be the best postures for falling asleep, so fibromyalgia sufferers continually shift and turn, trying to find the most comfortable arrangement of arms and legs. Such perpetual motion and adjustment can interrupt sleep. Finally, low levels of the brain chemical or *neurotransmitter* serotonin have been reported in people who have poor sleep patterns. Interestingly, serotonin is also documented in scientific studies to be low in people with fibromyalgia.[22-24] To understand how neurotransmitters work in the body, see Chapter 2.

❖ Altered Pain Perception

People with fibromyalgia experience a heightened sense of pain or hyperalgesia when exposed to normally mildly painful stimuli, and they consistently report feeling pain under typically non-painful conditions.[25, 26] Such sensing of supposedly non-painful events as painful is *allodynia*. High pain sensitivity and low pain thresholds are daily obstacles for people with fibromyalgia. The root of hyperalgesia and allodynia may be altered pain information processing in the brain and spinal cord of people with fibromyalgia.[27, 28] Specifically, certain brain chemicals or neurotransmitters may be to blame, such as serotonin, dopamine, or norepinephrine. These neurotransmitters are responsible for our body's interpretation of our environment, including painful or pleasurable stimuli, and our reactions to these interpretations. For example, the neurotransmitter serotonin sends the message to the brain that the chocolate cake you are eating is delicious. In contrast, norepinephrine is released when you are frightened or alarmed, prompting you to seek a safe place or to run from the danger.

Neurotransmitters are under increasing scrutiny by scientific investigators. In fact, in several studies, people with fibromyalgia were shown to have very different circulating levels of neurotransmitters compared to normal people.[29-32] For example, in people with fibromyalgia, neurotransmitters which decrease the body's attention and response to painful stimuli are blunted, and transmitters that send pain messages are overly active.[32] Thus, people with fibromyalgia actually interpret their surroundings differently than normal people, taking in information about their surroundings that many others comfortably ignore.[32, 33]

❖ Reynaud's Syndrome

Reynaud's Syndrome is an intolerance to cold that is felt chiefly in the extremities (hands, feet, fingers, toes) and is manifested by a blanching (turning white or blue) of the fingers and toes, usually accompanied by numbness and tingling. Then, the fingers are toes are quite painful as the numbness subsides and feeling returns to the extremities. Reynaud's can exist as an isolated disorder, but it frequently co-occurs with fibromyalgia.[34, 35] Researchers think that people with fibromyalgia who also have Reynaud's Syndrome have more abundant—or more sensitive—alpha-2 adrenergic receptors than people who do not experience these symptoms.

Alpha-2 adrenergic receptors are tiny docking stations located on cells in the body that bind to epinephrine (also called adrenaline). Epinephrine tells the blood vessels to contract or dilate, a response that is important when we experience cold or heat. Using epinephrine, our body can activate (turn on) alpha-2 receptors to constrict our blood vessels to keep heat inside our body, or the receptors can tell our blood vessels to dilate to let heat escape for cooling our body.

Thus, alpha-2 receptors are one way we respond to our environment, and having a receptor overabundance or oversensitivity might greatly enhance the body's responses to the environment...perhaps to a painful degree, as in Reynaud's Syndrome: the vessels constrict in response to cold, but they constrict so much that there is little circulation in the hands and feet, hence the blanching and numbness.

❖ Irritable Bowel Syndrome

Irritable bowel syndrome (IBS), which is defined as stomach pain, increased episodes of gas and bloating, along with changes in stool frequency and form[36] is commonly experienced by those with fibromyalgia.[37-40] In fact, most visits to bowel specialists or gastroenterologists are due to IBS, especially in people with fibromyalgia.[41, 42] Like Reynaud's Syndrome, IBS can occur in people who do not have fibromyalgia, and as such, it is a problematic stomach disorder all by itself. IBS is thought to be a hyperalgesia of the gut muscles and tissues (referred to as *viscera*), which is simply an increased attentiveness and heightened response to perceived pain in the gut.[42, 43] In fact, scientists speculate that the cause of IBS is tied to the cause of fibromyalgia because of these striking similarities in pain perception and processing.[44]

Characteristic IBS symptoms such as painful episodes or gas or changes in the stool might be a consequence of an individual's actions in response to the intense, stabbing pains of IBS. For example, sharp and sudden gut pains may promote unusual drinking or eating patterns such as gulping food and guzzling beverages to quell a rumbling stomach. Such rapid intake of nutrition can introduce more air into the gut. In contrast, not eating a meal all day and then consuming a large, heavy meal in the evening can overwhelm the gut and increase sensations of bloating and discomfort. Both actions can aggravate constipation or diarrhea, which are common aspects of IBS. Perhaps resolving the initial gut pain can bring about resolution of the other gastric symptoms, but these studies have yet to be conducted.

❖ Frequent Urination

People with fibromyalgia report needing to urinate more frequently than those who do not have fibromyalgia[45-49] Whether this phenomena is due to actual decreased bladder capacity is not clear, but the literature suggests that the feeling of needing to urinate frequently is tied to the altered perception of pain or pressure. Perhaps people with fibromyalgia may perceive that their bladder is full when it is almost empty and then interpret that sensation as an urge to urinate.

Either way, people with frequent urination problems state that not only do they need to urinate multiple times during the day, but also they awaken two or more times during the night to use the bathroom.[50] This problem is referred to as nocturia [*noct:* night, *uria:* urination]. Obviously, waking up frequently to urinate would fragment and disturb sleep, which could result in someone being tired the next morning. Moreover, after weeks and months of nocturia, persistent fatigue could be the result. Studies do not suggest that the sleep problems encountered in fibromyalgia are due to frequent urination; however, perhaps poor sleep quality allows someone to be awake enough to perceive that the bladder feels full.[50]

❖ Migraine

Migraine—also called a migraine headache—is common in fibromyalgia, and studies suggest that migraine headache and fibromyalgia are initiated by the same neurochemical events. Specifically, serotonin, which is implicated in fibromyalgia, may be important in migraine.[51, 52] Migraine is more than just a bad headache; it is a neurological disorder that is consistently experienced as a headache on one side of the head with a pulsing or throbbing aspect. Worse, people with fibromyalgia may suffer a more debilitating migraine than those who experience migraine without fibromyalgia.[53] Like fibromyalgia, migraine occurs in women more than in men, and Reynaud's Syndrome and migraine frequently occur together.[54] Likewise, migraine and IBS are reported to co-occur with fibromyalgia more so than other symptoms.[55]

❖ Paresthesias/Sensory Deficits

Numbness or paresthesia has been associated with fibromyalgia for more than 20 years.[6, 56-58] Paresthesias can be any tingling or numbness in the fingers or toes or they can be discrete patches of numbness on the skin, for example, a numb area on the back. The cause of these unusual areas of diminished or absent sensitivity is a mystery. Some scientists suggest that this phenomenon is a separate disease, not related to fibromyalgia, and is perhaps caused by demyelination, which is a destruction of the protective covering of the nerves.[59]

In contrast, in other studies including people with fibromyalgia, numbness was attributed to nerves taking longer to send a message, coupled with a longer muscle-response time after receiving a stimulus.[60] Other scientists think that the spinal cord, which transmits information about sensations, may be involved in numbness and tingling experienced by people with fibromyalgia. Irrespective of the origin or the reason, people with fibromyalgia do have abnormal sensory function with regard to temperature and pressure, so paresthesias may represent another area of peculiarity.[61-63] This topic will be covered more in Chapter 2 about fibromyalgia and diseases of the nerves.

❖ Drug Sensitivities

People with fibromyalgia are reported to have frequent unusual responses to drugs that are not intended consequences of drug therapy, and these atypical—but not harmful—responses are called side effects. Bad or harmful responses are referred to as adverse drug reactions.[64, 65] The reason for such unusual responses to medications is unclear. Perhaps sufferers of fibromyalgia are more inclined to try serious prescription, pain-relieving drugs—and to try more of them in a shorter period.[66] Taking multiple medications at once, referred to as *polypharmacy*, can have severe side effects in some susceptible populations.[67, 68] Alternately, people with fibromyalgia may be sensitive to medication as a direct consequence of their disorder, sensing side effects that might go unnoticed in normal individuals or interpreting general side effects as more harmful, adverse effects. For example, a drug side effect of mild—but tolerable—stomach-upset in a normal person may be felt as unrelenting nausea in a person with fibromyalgia. Presently, this phenomenon of unusual drug side effects is not well studied in the scientific literature.

In conclusion, the symptoms described here are those that most frequently co-occur with fibromyalgia. Of course, some people with fibromyalgia may have every symptom described here, and others may only have tender points and fatigue. Also, these additional symptoms may come and go. Fibromyalgia is such an individual experience that many variations may exist.

Early Ideas about Fibromyalgia

The word *fibromyalgia*, like many scientific and medical terms, has Greek or Latin roots, or both. Broken into its Greek and Latin roots, the word looks like this:

fibro   my   algia
Latin: fiber   Greek: muscle   Greek: pain

So, fibromyalgia literally means "a pain in the muscle fiber".

In the 1950's, before fibromyalgia was properly classified, fibromyalgia was known as *fibrositis*.[69, 70] Again, breaking the word into its roots, we find this:

fibro
Latin: fiber

sitis
Greek: inflammation

Thus, the choice of the term *fibrositis* suggests that physicians believed that inflammation was the source of the pain, and that they broadly classified fibrositis with other types of rheumatism, which is any inflammatory condition of the muscles or joints. As a consequence, aspirin-like compounds were recommended to reduce the purported inflammation and alleviate the symptoms.[71-73] To distinguish fibrositis from rheumatic disorders such as arthritis, physicians emphasized that fibrositis targeted the muscles and not the joints.[71, 74-77] Over time, scientific inquiry into the cause of fibromyalgia has revealed that inflammation is *not* a feature of the disease; therefore, the term fibrositis is no longer a correct way to refer to the condition.[56, 78, 79]

Also, since those early days, incredible new information has been discovered about fibromyalgia, including the prevalence of fibromyalgia (how many people have this problem), what may cause fibromyalgia, descriptions and reports about other associated symptoms of fibromyalgia, and information about diseases or disorders that may be confused with fibromyalgia. Also, as more research is being conducted to investigate the disease, new therapeutic strategies are being tested to alleviate the most common symptoms of fibromyalgia.

Who Has Fibromyalgia?

Research into fibromyalgia has increased significantly since the 1980's, when few articles describing fibromyalgia were published in the peer-reviewed scientific and medical literature, which is where scientists and physicians read about new diseases and treatments. In the 2000s, research (and publication of this research) in the literature has increased steadily (**Figure 2**). This surge in information and communication has allowed more people to be diagnosed with fibromyalgia and subsequently treated for its symptoms.

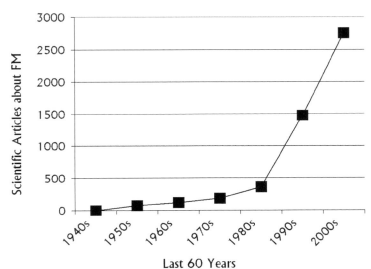

Last 60 Years

Figure 2 Peer-Reviewed, Scientific Literature about Fibromyalgia (FM) since 1940 (Source: PubMed)

From research and clinical studies, we now know that fibromyalgia might affect up to 2% of the US population.[80, 81] Scientists and physicians understand that these numbers reported in the scientific literature to describe people with fibromyalgia are likely *artificially low* because these reported values may only reflect two types of people. First, the numbers describe people who present to medical clinics with complaints of unrelenting pain and fatigue, who are then diagnosed with fibromyalgia. Second, the numbers describe people who are aware of their condition and who participate in fibromyalgia studies for new therapies. Thus, numerous people are not included in the present estimates of fibromyalgia prevalence because they are not aware that they have fibromyalgia. In addition, many people with fibromyalgia are aware of their condition, but they choose not to seek healthcare services for their fibromyalgia, so they are not counted.

In fact, some scientists and physicians suggest that fibromyalgia may be the 3rd most prevalent rheumatologic disease in the US.[82] Because of the historical considerations of fibromyalgia, which we discussed earlier, rheumatologists—physicians specializing in problems with the joints, muscles, tendons, and other connective tissues—are still routinely called upon to diagnose and treat fibromyalgia,[83] and the Arthritis Foundation is a major source of information and support for research into the disease.

Based upon the characteristics of those better-studied populations who do seek care or study participation, the scientific literature suggests that fibromyalgia is chiefly diagnosed in women 30 years-of-age and older.[80, 81, 84-86] Also, fibromyalgia has been documented in children, but these cases represent a minority in the scientific literature. Also, in children, both boys and girls are equally affected.[87-91] Because more adult women have fibromyalgia, scientists speculate that young boys "outgrow" fibromyalgia symptoms as they age, or that their symptoms are milder from the beginning. Either way, there appears to be a gender difference: girls are more greatly affected both in prevalence and in severity.[92] Chapter 7 describes what is currently known about fibromyalgia in children, which is referred to as *juvenile fibromyalgia*.

Investigators also suggest that the tendency to have fibromyalgia could be hereditary, because relatives of people with fibromyalgia are more likely to also have fibromyalgia.[87, 93, 94] Some researchers suggest that fibromyalgia is inherited as an *autosomal dominant* characteristic.[87, 95, 96] To understand what this means, you should remember that qualities we inherit from our parents are carried on chromosomes, of which there are two types. From our parents, we inherit *sex chromosomes* or *allosomes* and non-sex chromosomes or *autosomes*. Sex chromosomes are designated X (for female) and Y (for male). If you are female, you have two XX chromosomes (one X from your mother and one X from your father). If you are male, your chromosomes are X and Y (an X from your mother and a Y from your father). Thus, the father of a child determines whether that child is male or female.

Remaining chromosomes that do not determine whether we are male or female—autosomes (non-sex chromosomes)—carry information about additional characteristics such as right- or left-handedness, temperament, hair color, and other attributes. The gene variations carried on these chromosomes are *alleles*, specifically *autosomal alleles*. Alleles can be *dominant* or *recessive*. If the allele is dominant, it can override the traits carried on other alleles. For example, if the allele or gene set from our mother calls for us to have green eyes, and the allele from our father calls for us to have brown eyes, and we do indeed have brown eyes, then the brown eye allele is likely dominant. Thus, the green eye allele is probably recessive. Likewise, if you inherit a fibromyalgia allele from a parent and a normal allele from the other parent, you might still have fibromyalgia. This is because the allele for fibromyalgia dominates other alleles that call for being normal.

Although scientists believe that the overall predisposition for fibromyalgia is likely genetic, they also have considered whether a specific event may have triggered or initiated the fibromyalgia. This trigger may be environmental, such as a severe illness or an exposure to physical or psychological stresses such as a car accident or emotional distress, because people with fibromyalgia have frequently reported a childhood trauma.[93, 97-100] Alternately, fibromyalgia may not require a precipitating event such as a trauma or injury, and research into juvenile fibromyalgia is prompting people to investigate these types of questions and ideas. Chapter 2 of this book discusses what scientists and physicians understand at this time about the purported cause(s) of fibromyalgia.

Chapter Summary

- ❖ Fibromyalgia is a general but persistent pain throughout the whole body, especially the larger muscles, and this pain must be ongoing for 3 months or more, along with other symptoms.

- ❖ The pain can be burning or stinging, similar to the feeling of overused muscles.

- ❖ Fibromyalgia is clinically diagnosed by the presence of 11 of 18 tender points.

- ❖ Tender points may vary among people with fibromyalgia.

- ❖ Fibromyalgia includes non-muscular symptoms: fatigue, irritable bowel syndrome, frequent urination, unrefreshing sleep, numbness and tingling in the extremities, cold intolerance, headache, and drug sensitivities.

- ❖ People with fibromyalgia may have all of the muscular symptoms and none of the non-muscular concerns, or they may have a variety of the non-muscular problems in addition to pain and tenderness.

- ❖ Fibromyalgia was initially thought to be *fibrositis*, which is an inflammatory condition, so anti-inflammatory drugs were once thought to be helpful.

- ❖ Fibromyalgia is not due to inflammation; anti-inflammatory medications are generally ineffective.

- ❖ Fibromyalgia may affect 2% or more of the general population.

- ❖ Fibromyalgia chiefly affects women, but it has been diagnosed in men and in children.

- ❖ Fibromyalgia is probably hereditary, and it is likely a dominant characteristic, carried on a non-sex chromosome.

CHAPTER 2—WHAT CAUSES FIBROMYALGIA?

How Do We Classify Fibromyalgia?

As more research into fibromyalgia is completed and published, various ideas can be shared and compared about how people actually *acquire* fibromyalgia. For example, some researchers suggest that fibromyalgia is caused by infections, but support for this idea has been lacking in the scientific and medical literature.[101, 102] Other popular hypotheses (accepted explanations for observations) that have surfaced are as follows: fibromyalgia is an auto-immune disease; fibromyalgia is a disease that affects the nerves; or fibromyalgia is caused by a nervous system that does not function properly.[59, 103-110] This Chapter addresses each hypothesis about fibromyalgia, and provides evidence for or against each idea.

Is Fibromyalgia an Auto-Immune Disease?

Fibromyalgia has been thought to be an auto-immune disease (or a condition that precedes an auto-immune disease) because the symptoms of fibromyalgia are similar to those observed in other diseases which are known to be auto-immune in nature.[111], [112] To understand how fibromyalgia may or may not be a disease of auto-immunity, it is important to understand what an auto-immune disease *actually is.*

Under normal conditions, our bodies make antibodies to fight off invading and illness-producing viruses, bacteria, and other particles that enter our bodies through our nose, eyes, mouth, or skin. Often, our bodies will not only attack and destroy these particles but will also produce antibodies to these particles. Antibodies are chemicals that our bodies make to directly target these specific particles, latch onto them, and chew them up before they cause harm to us. These antibodies stay around in our bodies so that they can defeat particles that return. Because antibodies are specific for particular particles, pollen antibodies attack pollen particles that enter the body, and dog hair antibodies rush to obliterate invading dog hair particles. Laboratory tests can measure antibodies, and these tests can tell a physician what chemicals or particles a person has been exposed to and whether the exposure was recent.

Sometimes, the body creates antibodies that attack its very own cells. These antibodies are referred to as *auto-antibodies*—which are literally antibodies against the self. Auto-antibodies can be harmful if they attack healthy tissue in the body and destroy it. When the body continually manufactures auto-antibodies that destroy organs and other important tissues, an auto-immune disease may be responsible. In fact, with most auto-immune diseases, auto-antibodies can be found circulating in the body, and like other antibodies, these can be measured in laboratory tests. This finding is considered proof of an auto-immune condition, when other symptoms are present. Of course, because there is variation among people, some will have an auto-immune disease and lack detectable auto-antibodies, and many will have a positive test for auto-antibodies and still be healthy. Thus, a physician will weigh the evidence from many different sources to establish the diagnosis of an auto-immune disease.

Three well-studied auto-immune diseases are discussed next: arthritis, multiple sclerosis, and lupus erythematosus (simply referred to as lupus). These diseases—at first glance—are similar to fibromyalgia, but upon closer inspection, you will see that they are distinct diseases from fibromyalgia.

First, arthritis, specifically the rheumatoid type, is a painful condition in which the joints and connective tissues are assaulted by the body's own immune system, resulting in destruction of the cartilage that cushions the spaces between the bones. Rheumatoid arthritis, which is slightly different from osteoarthritis, is often confused with fibromyalgia because of the pain that is associated with it. Pain from arthritis comes from the cartilage damage that allows bones to rub together. Often, people will limit exercise because of arthritis, which makes the muscles weaker because they are not being used regularly. In extreme cases of arthritis, the cartilage destruction can cause the joints to bend or curve over time, so shoes and gloves do not fit properly, and activities like writing, driving, and cooking become difficult.

In rheumatoid arthritis, the presence of a rheumatoid factor auto-antibody can be measured in the blood. This factor is considered to be indicative of rheumatoid arthritis for most people (some people lack this factor).[113] Like other auto-antibodies, rheumatoid factor is made by the body to attack the body's joints, so it is no surprise that it can accumulate in the joints of many people who have rheumatoid arthritis, in addition to being present in the blood. Other auto-antibodies that can serve as markers of rheumatoid arthritis are under investigation.

Next, multiple sclerosis is an auto-immune disease that attacks the central nervous system. Like fibromyalgia, it affects women more than it affects men.[114] In multiple sclerosis, the body's own immune cells attack and destroy the outer coating of specific nerve cells or neurons. This nerve cell coating, referred to as *myelin*, behaves like the rubberized coating on electrical wire but, in addition to insulating the nerves much like rubber insulates copper wires, myelin also enables neurons to carry electrical messages throughout the body.

When myelin is damaged or missing from nerve cells, the neurons cannot conduct their signals properly, which can lead to vision loss, numbness, tingling, or dementia. Pain from multiple sclerosis is often felt in the back and in the limbs, and headaches are common for people with this disease.[115, 116] Also, in people with multiple sclerosis, two common auto-antibodies can be measured: anti-myelin oligodendrocyte glycoprotein and anti-myelin basic protein.[117, 118] The names of these auto-antibodies are not important for you to pronounce or remember. Rather, the idea to understand is that the body makes two auto-antibodies against myelin, which destroy the outer coating on nerve cells.

With lupus, myelin surrounding the nerve cells is destroyed as the body's immune cells attack the nerves. In addition, the body attacks major organs and produces inflammation in the heart, skin, liver, joints, lungs, blood vessels, and kidneys. Fatigue is a common consequence of lupus, and this auto-immune disease affects women more frequently than men.[119] There are many types of lupus, and many people diagnosed with lupus also meet the criteria for having fibromyalgia.[120]

Lupus patients have been reported to have several auto-antibodies when tested: antinuclear antibody, anti-DNA antibody, anti-Smith antibody, anti-phospholipid antibody, and anti-Ro and anti-La antibodies.[121] Once again, it is not important that you know what these antibodies do, but it is essential that you understand that the presence of these auto-antibodies is suggestive of lupus disease when considered with other lupus-like symptoms.

These auto-immune diseases are similar to fibromyalgia in that they disrupt the quality of life and cause diffuse pain; they seem to have no specific initiating event or cause; they can improve or worsen without much predictability; and all affect women more often than men.[122] In contrast, these auto-immune diseases are more destructive than fibromyalgia and can be disfiguring. Also, in fibromyalgia, the body does not destroy its own healthy tissue. No auto-antibodies have been detected in people with fibromyalgia, which provides additional evidence that auto-immunity is not a component of fibromyalgia.[123] Thus, at this time, fibromyalgia is not believed to be a disease of auto-immunity.[112, 124]

Is Fibromyalgia a Nerve Disorder?

Some scientists and physicians have considered that fibromyalgia might be a disorder of nerve transmission because some fibromyalgia symptoms such as paresthesias (tingling, numbness, and muscle weakness) are often caused by faulty nerve signaling.[59, 106] With some diseases, nerve signal-conduction errors can arise from disturbances within the nerve's myelin coating (see previous section about auto-immune diseases) or from disruptions in the nerve's environment, so nerve disorders have been proposed to explain the nerve-oriented symptoms of fibromyalgia. To understand how these ideas came about, one should first know how nerves behave when they are functioning properly.

Nerves, which are made of neurons or nerve cells, send messages all over the body in response to information processed from the environment. In normal individuals, nerves take in signals, send this information to the brain through the spinal cord, and receive interpretations from the brain to cause an action. This whole process happens in fractions of seconds. For example, the nerves of the fingers detect a hot stove top, and this message is sent to the brain, which replies with a second message to remove the fingers from the hot surface! These messages and interpretations rapidly occur throughout the day, and we are largely unaware of these processes until something goes wrong with them. A nerve problem or disorder is referred to as a *neuropathy* (*neuro:* nerve; *path:* disease).

The symptoms of fibromyalgia that are suggestive of a nerve disease are tingling or numbness felt in the fingers and toes and numb patches elsewhere on the body. Tingling and numbness typically means that nerves are being dangerously compressed, or they are not receiving information from nearby nerve-supporting cells so that they can do their job. This is a concern because nerves that fail to function properly over a period of time can die. Once neurons die, they cannot replace themselves. Dead nerves can be merely troublesome if they are critical to the health of a body part such as tooth or a fingernail. In those cases, the part that no longer receives nerve support may eventually decay and die (the tooth or nail may fall out), but the result is probably only cosmetically unattractive.

For nerves that communicate with major organs such as the skin, kidneys, or the heart, the results can be more devastating. For example, when nerves cannot communicate about the skin, injuries can go undetected and can worsen to the degree that an amputation maybe necessary. When nerves can no longer send critical signals to the kidneys or the heart, organ failure can result, which can be fatal. Thus, any symptoms that mimic a dangerous nerve disease or a neuropathy must be investigated.

To learn if actual neuropathies are responsible for altered sensations in people with fibromyalgia, scientists studied the skin nerves of people with fibromyalgia and found that they were slightly different when compared to skin nerves in normal people.[125-127] This idea is intriguing because through the nerves in our skin, we receive important information about our environment, which is then interpreted by the brain. Thus, people with fibromyalgia literally *feel* their environment differently than people who do not have fibromyalgia. These findings are surely interesting, but they are not sufficient to explain the overall sensitivity to pain that fibromyalgia brings.

Because fibromyalgia symptoms are felt not only on the skin (numbness, tingling, cold intolerance, increased sensation to painful stimuli), but are also experienced in muscles, scientists investigated whether the nerves in muscles are different between people with fibromyalgia and normal individuals. Using a microscope to view muscle samples from people with fibromyalgia, scientists observed a moth-eaten or ragged appearance of the muscle fibers, and this was not observed in muscle fibers of normal individuals.[128] Such a ragged appearance of muscle fibers can indicate a nerve injury or perhaps disease, although this was not proven to be the case in these particular studies.[129] This finding is exciting because it suggests that muscles of people with fibromyalgia are different at a microscopic level, compared to normal individuals.

Other studies have been conducted to investigate nerves that have motor (responsible for motion) and sensory (responsible for sensing the environment) functions in people with fibromyalgia. Researchers explored the idea that the nerves of people with fibromyalgia either improperly received messages about stimuli or inappropriately responded to these nerve signals. The results of these studies were not conclusive; no data proved that nerves of people with fibromyalgia were different with respect to the way they accepted or responded to signals.[60, 130]

Therefore, when all of these individual clinical findings are grouped and analyzed together, the idea of fibromyalgia being a disease of disordered nerves has minimal support.[110] So, the conclusion at this time is that additional studies are needed to provide evidence that disordered or damaged nerves are a feature of fibromyalgia. Presently, scientists do not believe that fibromyalgia is a nerve disorder.

Is Fibromyalgia an Altered Central Nervous System?

❖ Central Nervous System

Scientists are beginning to agree that fibromyalgia is a condition caused by a central nervous system that responds to the environment in a unique way: people with fibromyalgia experience every aspect of their surroundings differently than those who do not have fibromyalgia. Also, the bodies of people with fibromyalgia send messages that are not typical of normal people: reactions to normal stimuli are exaggerated and pain thresholds are significantly lower.

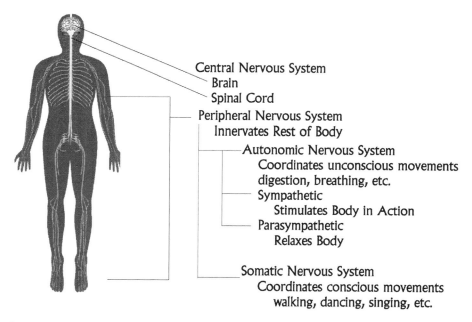

Figure 1. Human Nervous System and Components.

To understand whether the symptoms of fibromyalgia are caused by a central nervous system that is not performing normally or optimally, you should know something about the organization of the nervous system and what it does when it is functioning properly. First, you should know that the human nervous system is roughly divided into two components (**Figure** 1): the central nervous system, which is comprised of the brain and the spinal cord, and the peripheral nervous system. As the name implies, the peripheral nervous system handles the parts of the body which are more distant from the brain and spinal cord.

❖ Peripheral Nervous System

Then, the peripheral nervous system is further divided into two branches, the autonomic nervous system and the somatic nervous system. The autonomic nervous system handles the body's actions and movements that are not under our conscious control, such as breathing, digestion, and taking in information with our ears and eyes. These actions occur passively, without us doing anything; they are literally autonomic or automatic. Of course, we can influence their activity by holding our eyes open so that we do not blink or by holding our breath to control our respiration. We can only manipulate these systems for a short time, however. Then, the nervous system takes over again and regulates these processes.

The somatic nervous system manages our body's activities that are under our direct control, such as limb movement (typing, waving, running, dancing). The autonomic nervous system is divided again into parasympathetic and sympathetic divisions. The sympathetic side of the nervous system is stimulatory in nature—it increases the heart rate, enlarges structures deep in the lung so more air can enter, increases the size of the eye pupil so more light and information can enter the eye, diverts blood from the digestive system, and increases blood flow to the muscles. You can tell that these actions are similar: they are designed to help you move fast and stay alert.

The parasympathetic side of the nervous system opposes the sympathetic stimulatory effects—it decreases the heart rate, allows more blood to flow to the digestive system, makes branches of the lung smaller, and makes the eye pupil smaller. These processes are considered to be resting activities. When functioning normally, both the parasympathetic and sympathetic sides bring balance to the body, fine-tuning responses so that they are appropriate for the stimulus encountered.

❖ Neurotransmitters within the Nervous System

Within the nervous system, messages are carried by chemicals called neurotransmitters, which literally transmit neuron information. This process is initiated when a signal passes down a nerve fiber called an axon. This signal calls upon chemical neurotransmitters such as dopamine, acetylcholine, norepinephrine, or serotonin to be released into an area called the synapse. These specific neurotransmitters and their actions are discussed below. Once in the synapse, the neurotransmitter will bind to a special area called a receptor to initiate a second signal that will either promote or suppress an action. For example, the signal may prompt you to run because a bear is behind you, or the signal may make you stop running because you have reached a cliff!

Once the neurotransmitter does its job, the neurotransmitter is released from the receptor and can be taken back up into the nerve fiber that initially released it. This is called re-uptake. The longer the neurotransmitter stays in the synapse, the longer it can interact with receptors and send messages. Thus, if the re-uptake of a neurotransmitter is blocked, the neurotransmitter lingers in the synapse. This is the mechanism behind many drugs that target neurotransmission for disorders such as depression or bipolar disorder. Other drugs can manipulate neurotransmitters by actually inhibiting neurotransmitter release.

Each neurotransmitter may have a unique function, or its role may overlap or enhance the actions of other neurotransmitters. Serotonin is important in sleep and appetite regulation and can inhibit the sensation of pain. Norepinephrine constricts blood vessels and increases blood pressure along with stimulating anxiety, and it is reported to contribute to pain sensation. Dopamine is needed for perception of reality, daily movement, and sensing pleasurable activities. Interestingly, all of these neurotransmitters are also thought to be important in fibromyalgia.

So, the central nervous system, through an intricate process of neurotransmitter signaling by way of neurotransmission, is responsible for not only perceiving and discriminating among different stimuli. It is also in charge of informing the brain about the quality of the stimulus: is it painful and thus harmful, or is it pleasant and therefore likely not harmful. Through the central nervous system, you intercept signals and interpret that you are petting your neighbor's cat, which is fluffy and soft…or that you have put your hand on a stovetop that is hot and dangerous.

❖ Triggers for a Disordered Nervous System

Some researchers suggest that the heightened sense of pain associated with fibromyalgia arises from a disordered central nervous system that became disordered due to a one-time overwhelming illness or stress, either physical (such as a car accident) or psychological (such as domestic abuse).[131-133] Specifically, studies suggest a previous painful or destructive stimulus bombarded the body and the nervous system, which attuned it to harmful information.[110] Thus, physical or psychological trauma lowered the body's threshold for detecting pain, forever over-sensitizing it to normal sensations and interpreting these stimuli as sensations that must be avoided.[134-138]

In support of this idea, scientists conducted a small study with females and found that the study participants who had a history of more personal problems and various physically painful experiences also reported more symptoms of fibromyalgia.[139] Also, in studies of people with severely troubled childhoods (abuse, molestation, etc), chronic pain problems were more prevalent in that group than in people who had generally happy childhoods.[140-143]

In contrast, studies including subjects with whiplash injury were found to have no greater tendency to have fibromyalgia than people who did not sustain such an injury.[144] Such differences between these findings might be explained by the fact that one study included trauma from a variety of sources that had both physical and psychological effects—such as abuse—and the other study included only one physical injury that was sustained through a single event—such as a car wreck. Perhaps traumas must be multiple and ongoing, with a significant psychological component, to permanently alter the central nervous system. Likewise, studies including children with fibromyalgia appear to be in contrast with the trauma-as-a-trigger theory: children with fibromyalgia did not report experiencing events which might have initiated their fibromyalgia.[145] Thus, the data are divided on the idea that trauma predisposes the individual to fibromyalgia.

An idea worth considering is that people with fibromyalgia have a greater tendency to recall more vividly painful past events due to the way a person with fibromyalgia processes such events—more sensitively and with a lower threshold for unpleasantness. Thus, these episodes would be magnified and more memorable. In contrast, normal individuals might not recall or report every past trauma because it was not given too much import. Either way, people with fibromyalgia are sensorially unique, so additional studies to investigate this idea are warranted.[146-150]

❖ No Trigger Required for a Disordered Nervous System

In support of findings that trauma or a trigger is not necessary for fibromyalgia, some scientists have suggested that fibromyalgia is just a novel or unusual state of being for an individual.[151] Perhaps people with fibromyalgia just process pain differently than normal individuals.[152] Thus, people with fibromyalgia are considered hypervigilant and hyperalgesic.[107-110] *Hypervigilant* refers to people who have a greater than normal wariness or watchfulness. Hypervigilant people are more acutely aware of themselves and their environment; they notice sounds and movements that normal people tune out. As we mentioned in the previous chapter, someone who is hyperalgesic is extremely sensitive to pain and will report feeling pain from normally non-painful stimuli.[149, 153-155] For most people, there is a balance between pain-sensing and pain-blocking components of the central nervous system, and this harmony helps regulate and normalize responses to the environment. In people with fibromyalgia, this balance could be shifted such that the pain-sensing features are turned up and the pain-blocking aspects are turned down.[156]

Because pain is a unique experience that depends on interpretation by an individual's central nervous system, people will vary in their perception of pain and in their response to pain. To understand the differences among people and their experience of noxious (harmful, painful) stimuli, you could line up everyone on the planet, based on their sensitivity to pain. Along this line, you could position those people with high pain thresholds on one end of the line or spectrum. Normal responders to pain would be grouped in the middle, and they would comprise the largest group of people. Then, people who are sensitive to pain would be grouped at the other end of the spectrum, on the opposite side of those who have high pain thresholds. Then, next to the pain-sensitive individuals, you could position the people who have fibromyalgia.

See **Figure 2** for an example of this type of spectrum or "scale". Such differences in perception and response to pain could suggest that the central nervous system of people with fibromyalgia is likely different from that of everyone else on the planet, and groups of people with fibromyalgia are likely similar to one another. Such an idea is helpful in unraveling the reasons why specific additional symptoms are commonly found in fibromyalgia patients such as IBS, migraine, increased need for urination, and others, and why these symptoms have common threads.

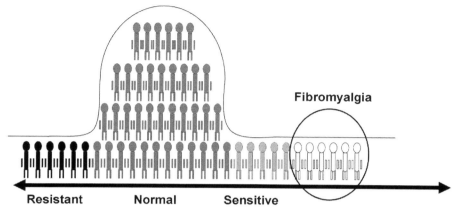

Figure 2. People Grouped by Their Ability to Perceive Pain.

Clearly, every part of the body can be hypersensitive in people with fibromyalgia, so it would be reasonable to assume that some relatively normal sensations in the gut, such as hunger or gastric irritation, could be perceived as painful for someone who is ultra sensitive to pain. Likewise, the sensation of a barely full bladder would be interpreted as a strong urge to urinate by someone with low thresholds for pain. Also, a hard-backed chair could be felt as an unyielding, uncomfortable place to sit for a person with fibromyalgia, and a belt that is cinched a little tighter than normal around the waist might be interpreted as an unrelenting squeezing sensation around one's middle. These additional symptoms—which have common links—are discussed in detail in the following Chapters.

Detecting Fibromyalgia

Experts in science and medicine agree that fibromyalgia is a unique disorder, but there is no reliable diagnostic marker, referred to as a biomarker, to distinguish people who have fibromyalgia from people who are not afflicted—other than subjective complaints [See below]. Thus, fibromyalgia is difficult to confirm. Proving the presence of fibromyalgia may not be a great concern for those who have it and have found ways to manage it quietly, but lacking reliable proof is disastrous for others. Imagine the difficulty of explaining to an employer that you are ill with nonspecific symptoms that come and go unexpectedly. Moreover, envision the frustration for someone seeking disability status because this invisible affliction is so severe that he cannot perform his job. In fact, the lack of a proper diagnostic reference or "proof" for fibromyalgia has led some judges and juries who hear disability lawsuits to deny the claims of fibromyalgia sufferers because the disease cannot be "seen".[157, 158]

❖ Reliable Laboratory Tests

Thus, a definitive and reliable test for fibromyalgia is needed to determine the presence or severity of the disorder. For example, the presence of the hormone beta human chorionic gonadotropin [β-HCG] in a woman's blood, which can be measured in a routine laboratory test, is accepted to be evidence that the woman is pregnant. This is because β-HCG is made and secreted by the developing embryo [in rare cases β-HCG is secreted by tumors, but this is rare enough to be set aside for this comparison]. In contrast, the absence of β-HCG in a woman's blood is considered to be evidence that she is *not* pregnant [or that her pregnancy is too early to be detected]. Also, higher β-HCG values in women can correlate to pregnancies that are further along. So, the β-HCG laboratory test has the power to detect a specific condition, and it can reflect the degree, progression, or severity of the condition. Unfortunately, a laboratory test to provide evidence for the presence of fibromyalgia, much less the severity of it, does not exist at this time.[82, 159] Scientists have begun looking for a biomarker much like the laboratory test described above, and the information below describes some of this work to date.

❖ Biomarkers for Fibromyalgia

Within the nervous system, neurotransmitters are the actual messengers of information, and these are of enormous interest to scientists who study fibromyalgia. Neurotransmitters travel through nerve cells or through nervous tissue and tell the brain about stimuli, and then they help the body respond to the stimuli. Also intriguing is the finding that people with fibromyalgia have lower levels of specific neurotransmitters such as serotonin. Serotonin has anti-depressant effects in the brain—it is secreted in the body in response to certain pleasing stimuli such as eating delicious food like cake, pasta, bread, or chocolate—and in people with depression, serotonin is reported to be low.[150, 160-163] Interestingly, the finding that serotonin is low in fibromyalgia sufferers might indicate that sufficient serotonin is not made for the body to feel good, or that the chronic pain of fibromyalgia depresses serotonin production. In light of this finding, some scientists have suggested that drugs that increase the amount of serotonin circulating in our bodies might be a good therapy for fibromyalgia. These drugs are discussed in Chapter 4.

Another feel-good neurotransmitter with natural analgesic properties is dopamine, and this chemical is reported to be low in people with fibromyalgia.[164, 165] Scientists think that long-term stress such as that produced by chronic and unrelenting pain may suppress dopamine production.[33, 166] Another view is that low dopamine levels in individuals may actually produce the symptoms of fibromyalgia.[165, 167] Determining which came first—low dopamine and then the onset of fibromyalgia, or fibromyalgia symptoms which eventually depressed dopamine—is a goal of future studies, especially because dopamine and serotonin are crucial neurotransmitters which participate in events all over the body, from the gut to the brain.

Other neurochemicals are of interest in fibromyalgia studies.[32, 146] For example, norepinephrine, the *fight-or-flight* neurotransmitter, is high in people with fibromyalgia compared to normal people.[149] This could mean that the stress of chronic pain causes these individuals to overproduce norepinephrine, which keeps these individuals ever vigilant for additional painful stimuli, or that people with fibromyalgia have too much norepinephrine in the first place, which causes the hypervigilance and hyperalgesia. In clinical studies, blockade of this neurotransmitter was shown to decrease pain in persons with fibromyalgia symptoms, and injection of norepinephrine caused the pain to return.[149] Thus, low serotonin, low dopamine, and high norepinephrine are implicated as a biomarker for fibromyalgia but because these very transmitters are also abnormal in other disorders, they are not specific enough at this time to be diagnostic for fibromyalgia alone: a different biomarker is needed.

Cytokines, which are chemicals that circulate in the body to interpret pain signals have been reported to be high in fibromyalgia sufferers. In particular, specific cytokines that are increased in people with fibromyalgia are interleukins and tumor necrosis factors—specific chemicals that are released by our body which influence our perception of pain. These cytokines are not thought to be the *actual source* of the pain experienced in fibromyalgia, rather they are just proof that the body is receiving a pain signal.[168] Intriguingly, other studies have not supported the findings of high levels of cytokines.[169] Thus, these are not reliable biomarkers for fibromyalgia at this time.

Insulin-like growth factor, a chemical similar to insulin (which tells the body to store sugar), was shown to be lower in people with fibromyalgia, compared to people who did not have fibromyalgia. Insulin-like growth factor is released in the body in response to growth hormone, and it helps the body regulate cell growth and development, especially that of nerve cells. Thus, researchers believed that giving growth hormone to people with fibromyalgia would increase insulin-like growth factor and improve the health of nerve cells, and these researchers did report that adding growth hormone to fibromyalgia therapy had modestly positive results.[170] In contrast, another research group did not find differences in insulin-like growth hormone in people with fibromyalgia, and they did not recommend that growth hormone would be effective.[171] Thus, the role of insulin-like growth factor in fibromyalgia is not clear at this time.

People with fibromyalgia were also reported to have less ghrelin, a hormone made in the stomach and pancreas (and in the hypothalamus, where it calls for the release of growth hormone). Ghrelin increases appetite by detecting low energy stores, telling the body to consume food. Thus, ghrelin is high before a meal and decreases after a meal in normal individuals. The relevance of ghrelin to fibromyalgia symptoms is not presently clear.[171] If low ghrelin contributes to the pain that often accompanies hunger—a pain that might be more easily ignored in healthy people—perhaps ghrelin-mediated hunger pangs are grossly magnified in individuals with fibromyalgia, replicating gastric distress.

Other interesting results that may have relevance after further investigation include the finding of lower levels of certain antioxidants (chemicals that protect the cells in the body from oxidants that can damage tissues) in people with fibromyalgia. However, measuring antioxidants is difficult, and often just measuring these compounds in the clinic alters their status.[172] Presently, antioxidant measurement is not useful for assessing fibromyalgia.

A group of scientists discovered that the novel neuromodulator, Substance P, is higher in the cerebrospinal fluid of people with fibromyalgia. [173-175] Substance P is a neuropeptide—a compound made of several small organic molecules called amino acids—that travels within nerve cells to communicate information, specifically information about pain. Thus, the finding that Substance P—a modulator of pain—is higher in fibromyalgia sufferers is very interesting and warrants further investigation.

Fibromyalgia presents itself to different people in various ways, and the full range of fibromyalgia sufferers may not fit neatly into groups previously studied in clinical settings.[176] So, it would be reasonable that not all sufferers would respond to therapies or treatments in the same manner that clinical study groups might respond.[177-179] Moreover, as more people are identified with fibromyalgia, more information will be collected from them. These findings will inform new studies into mechanisms of fibromyalgia and the best treatments for the symptoms.

Chapter Summary

- ❖ Fibromyalgia has been proposed to be an auto-immune disease and a disease in which nerves are damaged. Minimal evidence supports these proposals at this time.

- ❖ Studies suggest that fibromyalgia is due to a disordered nervous system that causes errors in an individual's ability to perceive pain and process information about that pain, but these studies are not complete.

- ❖ Scientists agree that the central nervous system of people with fibromyalgia is unique.

- ❖ Scientists are divided on the idea that a specific trigger or trauma is needed to bring about fibromyalgia symptoms.

- ❖ People can be categorized by sensitivity to pain or perception of pain, and people with fibromyalgia appear to be at the extreme end of this categorization.

- ❖ At this time, no clinical laboratory test can definitively label people with fibromyalgia.

- ❖ In clinical assessments, people with fibromyalgia have been shown to have abnormal levels of neurotransmitters (serotonin, norepinephrine, dopamine), and they have increased amounts of substances that transmit pain messages such as Substance P.

CHAPTER 3—
DISORDERS SIMILAR
TO FIBROMYALGIA

As fibromyalgia research increases and more of this information becomes available in the scientific and lay press about the disorder, we learn more about conditions similar to fibromyalgia. In fact, people who are eventually diagnosed with fibromyalgia report that they are frequently tested for many of these diseases and disorders as their physician sorts out the problem, eliminating other causes for the fatigue, pain, etc. Because these diseases or syndromes may be confused with fibromyalgia, each condition is described and compared to fibromyalgia.

❖ Chronic Fatigue Syndrome

As more people reported pain and fatigue to their physicians and sought treatment for these problems, the medical community began gathering information to suggest that fibromyalgia was similar to another disorder, chronic fatigue syndrome (CFS). In fact, patients who sought care for CFS were found to have many symptoms of fibromyalgia—sleep disorders, depressiveness, multiple tender points, and generalized body pain.[180-182] This lead some physicians to suggest that fibromyalgia was actually a facet or subsyndrome of CFS.

At this time, we know that CFS and fibromyalgia are distinct medical conditions. CFS is characterized by a constant generalized fatigue that lasts greater than 6 months and that typically begins like the flu. CFS may include muscular pain.[181] Fibromyalgia, which is characterized by the presence of persistent and often debilitating pain, is considered to be more of a burden than CFS.[183] Many clinicians initially believed that CFS was brought on by the Epstein-Bar virus, a type of herpes virus.[184] However, subsequent scientific and clinical studies have not concluded that this virus is the cause of CFS.[185, 186]

❖ Depression

Depression is a mental state in which a person feels unhappy or pessimistic, moods that can be complicated by feelings of anxiety, rage, guilt, or despair. These feelings can lead the person with depression to decline full participation in activities of daily living such as socializing, working, eating, or bathing. Depression is characterized by fatigue, restless sleep, back pain, headaches, and lack of ability to concentrate.[187, 188] These physical symptoms, which can diminish the enjoyment of life are present in almost 75% of those with depression.[189] Likewise, people with fibromyalgia experience similar suffering that can disrupt their quality of life.[190] Often, depression and fibromyalgia are reported to occur together in an individual.[191, 192] What is not well understood is whether the fibromyalgia was a factor in bringing about the depression or if depression measurements are simply not sensitive enough to distinguish depressive symptoms from those arising from fibromyalgia alone.[193, 194] Interestingly, depression is associated with abnormal levels of the neurotransmitters serotonin, norepinephrine, and dopamine, which regulate the body's response to stress and influence emotions, patterns of sleep, and appetite. Thus, many antidepressant medications regulate the amount of these neurotransmitters to restore normal neurotransmitter levels. Similar medications have been investigated for fibromyalgia with differing outcomes.[195-198]

❖ Arthritis

Arthritis, specifically rheumatoid arthritis, affects about 1.3 million adults.[199, 200] Osteoarthritis, which is also referred to as *degenerative arthritis*, is thought to be a problem for about 27 million US residents.[199, 200] Arthritis is similar to fibromyalgia in that pain may be felt throughout the body, and often people who suffer from arthritis report stiffness in their limbs in the morning after rising, which is a feature of fibromyalgia.[3] However, unlike fibromyalgia, arthritis is felt in the joints, whereas fibromyalgia is restricted to muscles. Also, interestingly, arthritis affects men and women equally—and can affect children—but fibromyalgia, which also affects men and children, chiefly affects women.[201] Fatigue may accompany arthritis, if it disrupts the quality and duration of restful sleep. Arthritis is covered in more detail in Chapter 2.

❖ Myofascial Pain Syndrome

Myofascial pain syndrome involves a more focused type of pain than the diffuse or wide-spread pain experienced in fibromyalgia.[202, 203] The term *myofascial* simply refers to the site of the pain (*myo:* muscle; *fascia:* connective tissue). Myofascial pain syndrome is thought to arise from overuse of muscles,[204] and it is characterized by the presence of *trigger points*, which are taut areas of muscle that are painful when pressure is directly applied.[205-207] Also, in myofascial pain syndrome, the muscles are often described as "ropy" and their tightness results in a decreased range of motion for the individual experiencing it.[208] In contrast to trigger points which are more discrete areas of pain, the tender points associated with fibromyalgia are areas of widespread tenderness in the muscle, where the muscle meets a tendon, in the cushiony area (referred to as the bursa) where a bone meets a tendon, or where fat covers a bony area (fat pad).[205] Because tender points can occur in the bursa, fibromyalgia has been confused with bursitis or tendinitis.[209]

❖ Generalized Myalgia

Myalgia or chronic muscle pain can arise from various sources such as simply repeatedly injuring a muscle, or the myalgia can be a result of something more severe such as scoliosis, which is a curvature of the spine that affects the supporting muscles and ligaments. Also, general joint looseness (referred to as *joint laxity*) can make the surrounding muscles work harder to sustain posture and activities. Iron or Vitamin D deficiency can cause muscle pain, and hypothyroidism (underactive thyroid, see below for more information) can result in myalgia. Muscles can ache because of viruses that cause influenza, the common cold, or pneumonia. If you suspect that your muscle aches are due to viral issues, you should visit a physician to confirm this, and to ensure that you manage your viral illness properly. As disturbing as myalgias can be, correcting the underlying problem that led to the myalgia, if possible, often reverses the painful condition.[204]

❖ Carpal Tunnel Syndrome

Carpal Tunnel Syndrome is characterized by pain, weakness, numbness, and tingling in the hands that is noticed when the wrist is flexed or extended. This pain and loss of sensation is caused by increased pressure in the nerves in the wrist, specifically the intracarpal canal.[210] Often, carpal tunnel syndrome is caused by repetitive stresses that may occur on the job, such as in professions which involve typing, computer keyboarding, and other technical jobs involving hand-tools which require the same hand and arm motions to be made continuously.[211, 212] The numbness or weakness in the hands in fibromyalgia can be confused with carpal tunnel and Reynaud's Syndrome, the latter of which is distinguished by numbness in the hands and fingers in response to cold. Because carpal tunnel is restricted to the wrists and hands, this condition is not difficult to differentiate from fibromyalgia-related issues.

❖ Gout

Gout is a metabolic disease characterized by recurrent episodes of acute arthritis, which arises from the painful accumulation of uric acid crystals in the joints. [213] A person with gout cannot break down or metabolize uric acid, which collects in cartilage of the joints and tendons, causing inflammation, joint swelling, stiffness, and severe pain.[214, 215] Uric acid is formed in the body from normal body processes that involve the amino acid purine, which is found in high quantities in some meats and sea foods. In normal individuals, the uric acid is excreted from the body. With gout, uric acid is not excreted, perhaps due to a defect in the kidney which excretes most of the body's burden of uric acid.[216] Because gout attacks the joints, the areas of pain are different from those observed in fibromyalgia.

❖ Sciatica

Sciatica is a painful condition caused by compression or irritation of the sciatic nerve or a set of nerves that eventually branch into the sciatic nerve. The sciatic nerve is the longest and widest nerve in the body, originating in the lower back and running down into the buttock, continuing on within the leg.[217] The pain that arises from such nerve compression or irritation is felt in the lower back, buttocks, legs, and perhaps as far as the feet.[217, 218] Sometimes, in severe cases of sciatica, numbness and weakness occur. Some people find it difficult to stand or walk when they have sciatic pain. Interestingly, when sciatica occurs, it may affect only one side of the body. Sciatica is similar to fibromyalgia in that the symptoms may arise for no apparent reason, but the pain of fibromyalgia is more evenly distributed, occurring on both sides of the body. Like fibromyalgia, there are no optimal treatments for sciatica, and the ultimate reason for the nerve compression or irritation is important in the treatment plan. For example, a herniation of the spine discs can give rise to sciatic nerve compression and pain.[219] Many experts believe that sciatica can be induced from sitting for long durations. Often, removing the source of nerve compression or irritation is curative for many people with sciatica.

❖ Hypothyroidism

The thyroid is gland located inside your neck and produces calcitonin, a compound which tells your body how to handle calcium, and two thyroid hormones (thyroxine and tri-iodothyronine, which are referred to as T-4 and T-3, respectively). T-4 and T-3 tell your body how to process fat and carbohydrates and regulate your body temperature among other functions. An underactive thyroid causes *hypothyroidism,* which simply means low thyroid activity. Hypothyroidism can produce symptoms much like those experienced in fibromyalgia. Fatigue, weakness, weight gain, cold intolerance, muscle cramps, muscle aches, constipation, and other symptoms are all indicators of a thyroid that is not performing as it should.

Hypothyroidism can occur after certain auto-immune diseases, after treatment for an overactive thyroid (hyperthyroidism), after thyroid surgery, or because of some drug treatments. Sometimes, hypothyroidism can be a problem after a pregnancy or due to an iodine deficiency. To know whether your fatigue and muscle aches are due to either fibromyalgia or hypothyroidism, you can have a thyroid function test to determine if the thyroid is causing your symptoms. If so, drugs can be prescribed to alleviate the symptoms caused by thyroid malfunction and restore adequate levels of thyroid hormones.

❖ Lyme Disease

Lyme disease is an infectious disease caused by bacteria, specifically, *Borrelia burgdorferi* in the US (other forms may cause other Lyme diseases in other countries) which is carried by ticks which then transmit the disease to humans through tick bites. Like fibromyalgia, Lyme disease can cause headache, fatigue, and depression,[220, 221] but unlike fibromyalgia, these symptoms are often accompanied by a fever and a characteristic bull's-eye or target-shaped skin rash. Without proper and timely antibiotic treatment, Lyme disease can affect the joints, heart, and nervous system. Often, even with treatment, the fatigue, problems with sleep, and issues with cognition persist.[221] Frequently, Lyme disease an initial illness that is ruled out by a physician when assessing symptoms of fibromyalgia.[222, 223]

❖ Sprains, Strains, and Other Pains

Physical injury can contribute to achiness and stiffness that mimics the pain of fibromyalgia. Sprains and strains are generally attributed to accidental muscle trauma or unintentional overuse. In contrast, the soreness often experienced from deliberate physical exertion is called delayed onset muscle soreness (DOMS). DOMS is usually experienced the day after intense exercise. Unlike fibromyalgia, DOMS dissipates over a few days, and many people find that "working through", the pain by engaging in moderate exercise, is helpful. Also, over-the-counter analgesics and anti-inflammatory medications are excellent for relieving the pain of DOMS, sprains, and strains. Symptoms experienced in fibromyalgia do not go away after a few days, and they usually discourage people from participating in exercise at all. As tough as a sprain or muscle strain may be until the tissue heals, these injuries are easy to distinguish from fibromyalgia because we can usually recall the event or the exercise that precipitated the pain.

❖ Drug-related Muscular Pain

Often, drugs can produce myalgias, or muscles pains. Colchicine is one such drug. People notice that after discontinuing the suspected drug, the pain disappears rapidly. Statins, which are widely prescribed for lowering cholesterol, can also cause muscle pain, and in rare cases, statins can cause a severe muscle damage called *rhabdomyolysis*, which is a condition in which muscle cells break down and are excreted from the body through the urine. A dark, cola-colored urine is an indicator of this problem. Of course, as with all unusual muscle symptoms that arise after starting a new drug therapy, you should contact your prescribing physician and share your concerns to protect your health.

Evaluating Fibromyalgia

From the scientific literature, we know that people with fibromyalgia experience and process painful sensations differently than people who do not have fibromyalgia.[33, 224] We also know that, quite possibly, the entire central nervous system of people with fibromyalgia is unique.[33] Also, we understand that the perception of pain is an individual characteristic, so fibromyalgia may affect different people in unique ways, and the severity of symptoms may be drastically different among individuals with fibromyalgia for these reasons.

❖ The Fibromyalgia Impact Questionnaire [The FIQ]

Because of this variety in the fibromyalgia experience, clinicians and scientists saw the need for a standardized system of questions, the answers to which were indicative of the severity of fibromyalgia. From this need, the Fibromyalgia Impact Questionnaire—or the FIQ—was developed in the 1980s by clinicians. The FIQ has been modified and improved over time, and presently, the FIQ has been translated into more than 8 languages.[225, 226]

The FIQ, which you can take and score for yourself for free at the following link: http://www.myalgia.com/FIQ/Bennett%20FIQ%20review.pdf, is a good initial approach to learn more about the range of symptoms that are considered to be authentic for assessing fibromyalgia. The core of the questionnaire focuses on larger muscles. Less emphasis is given to smaller muscles, such as those in the hands.

This accurately reflects the scientific consensus for fibromyalgia symptoms—that the larger muscle groups are most affected.

The questionnaire takes 3–5 minutes for most people to complete because the instructions are easy to follow and the questions are straight-forward. The FIQ seems to be unbiased. This means that you can measure fibromyalgia symptoms accurately irrespective of your race, occupation, economic status, and education.[225] So, no group has an advantage in the FIQ, and scores do not favor certain lifestyles. Such features allow everyone to evaluate fibromyalgia symptoms confidently.

The typical fibromyalgia patient will score 50 on the FIQ, and the more impaired fibromyalgia patient will report values of 70 and higher.[225] The FIQ can be used repeatedly over a period of time, and the scores can be compared to assess improvement or worsening of fibromyalgia symptoms. In fact, the FIQ is used multiple times to measure the benefit of experimental drug therapy in clinical trails for fibromyalgia, and the FIQ is sensitive enough to show changes in symptoms. Also, the FIQ is specific; it can detect true fibromyalgia symptoms and distinguish these from other related pain disorders.[225]

Accessing Information about Fibromyalgia

The FIQ is just one piece of information that you can access to learn more about fibromyalgia. Additional literature or scientific reports about fibromyalgia are easy to obtain but difficult to find! That paradox is easily explained by emphasizing that the information is out there, but it is easier to find if you know exactly where to look.

❖ The National Library of Medicine (The NLM)

There are numerous portals or windows through which professionals and nonprofessionals can share, find, and access information about fibromyalgia, or any disease or condition. The best-known access point is probably The National Library of Medicine (NLM), which is the world's largest scientific/medical literature repository.

The NLM is physically located at the National Institutes of Health (NIH) in Bethesda, Maryland. The NIH, in addition to having staff scientists who conduct research into human health and disease prevention, also awards grant money to US scientists outside the NIH for basic science and clinical research. At the NIH, the NLM seeks and collects biomedical healthcare and technology resources and information. Presently, the NLM has more than 9 million items in its collection, which includes manuscripts, journals, reports, microfilms, images, and rare medical literature. The NLM collections can be viewed online at http://www.nlm.nih.gov/. Through NLM, one can access—for free—various databases including PubMed, which is an NLM service featuring more than 17 million citations from Medline (http://medlineplus.gov) and other life science journals for biomedical articles that date as far back as 1949.

If you cannot find this information on your own using a computer and online connection, your public library will likely have a computer for you to use, and librarians can provide assistance for accessing information online. Librarians are magnificent sources for both online help and instruction in acquiring literature.

Abstracts, which are summaries of research papers, are usually free through PubMed or other online indexing services. The full articles may cost a few dollars or a subscription may be required. Thus, abstracts of scientific and medical articles are often easier to obtain than the full, published pieces. Abstracts are synopses or summaries of the purpose or goals of the study and the conclusions. Because scientific and medical journals are specialty subjects, subscriptions can be as much as a hundred dollars for one year. Some medical universities subscribe their library system to the journal, and by using their computers, you may be able to access the articles at no cost. Often free online registration is the only necessity for gaining access. Also, you can copy the article from the paper or hard copy version of the journal if your medical university library carries the subscription. Ask a librarian for the best approach to finding what you need.

❖ The Scientific Literature

Articles [and abstracts of these articles] that you find in the scientific literature about fibromyalgia are different from articles written for newspapers or magazines. The information contained in scientific papers is collected, analyzed, and reported under a rigorous peer-review system before it is published. Peer-review is a scientific procedure in which researchers report the details of their experiments or studies in the form of a manuscript and submit it to a medical or scientific journal. Once the paper is received at the journal, journal editors send the manuscript for review by experts in the particular area of expertise covered in the paper. Expert reviewers are other scientists or clinicians who evaluate the work in the paper and either recommend that the journal accept the paper and publish it, or they recommend that the journal accept the paper only after the author has made particular revisions to the paper. Alternatively, the expert reviewer can recommend that the journal reject the paper and not publish it at all. This type of oversight is the hallmark of good science, and all peer-reviewed scientific papers go through this process before being published and shared with the scientific and medical community. Because of this rigor and reliability in the communication of science and medicine, professionals in these fields agree that the peer-reviewed published literature is the first and best source of information about diseases, drugs, research, and related topics. In contrast "scientific information" appearing in non-scientific, non-peer-reviewed publications cannot always be guaranteed, and such information may pose more harm than help.

To supplement information about fibromyalgia that you find online or in the library, you can select articles from the bibliography of this book. To do this, find the citation (superscript number in the text) near the text you most want to learn more about, and then turn to the Bibliography or reference section of this book. The authors of the article are listed first, followed by the title of the article, the journal in which the article appears, and then the year, volume, issue (if any), and pages are listed. You can find these articles using a search engine on the Internet or you can have a librarian find or order the article for you.

Chapter Summary

- ❖ Many disorders share similarities with fibromyalgia.

- ❖ Chronic fatigue syndrome, which may be a subsyndrome of fibromyalgia, often has a sudden onset is characterized by fatigue and sleep disorders and muscle soreness.

- ❖ Depression shares many symptoms with fibromyalgia, and depression is common in people with fibromyalgia.

- ❖ Arthritis produces stiffness and pain like fibromyalgia but this pain is due to inflammation; is limited to joints; and is destructive or disfiguring.

- ❖ Myofascial pain syndrome involves pain of the muscles or connective tissues from muscle overuse, and it is characterized by painful trigger points and "ropy" muscles.

- ❖ Generalized myalgia is not as long-lasting as fibromyalgia and has many origins.

- ❖ Carpal tunnel syndrome differs from fibromyalgia in that the wrists and arms are targeted, whereas fibromyalgia is felt over most of the body.

- ❖ Gout is a type of arthritis caused by painful accumulation of uric acid crystals in the joints and must be controlled with diet and medications.

- ❖ Sciatica, caused by a compressed or irritated nerve, mimics the pain of fibromyalgia because it arises suddenly and may be focused in the back, buttocks, and legs, but alleviating the source of the irritation can be curative.

❖ Hypothyroidism or underactive thyroid can cause muscle soreness and fatigue but a laboratory test can affirm hypothyroidism as the source of the symptoms, and corrective medications can be prescribed.

❖ Lyme disease from tick bites can produce headaches, fatigue, and pain, but clinical assessment along with a typical rash can rule out fibromyalgia as the cause of the symptoms.

❖ Sprains, strains, and other pains from minor injuries can cause achiness and stiffness like fibromyalgia, but this pain usually subsides in a short time and analgesics effectively control pain.

❖ Drugs can cause muscle pain, but the pain goes away after the drug is discontinued.

❖ Fibromyalgia can be measured with the Fibromyalgia Impact Questionnaire (FIQ).

❖ A score of 50 on the FIQ is typical of most people with fibromyalgia.

❖ Reliable information about fibromyalgia and new treatments for this disease can be accessed from a library or through the world-wide web, via online sites.

❖ Medical and scientific information about fibromyalgia should be from reliable and tested sources, preferably peer-reviewed scientific or medical literature.

Chapter 4—Drugs Used to Treat Fibromyalgia

Approved Drugs for Fibromyalgia

Recently three new drugs have been approved by the US Food and Drug Administration (FDA) for use in treating fibromyalgia—pregabalin (Lyrica), milnacipran (Savella), and duloxetine (Cymbalta).[197, 227-232] These three prescription drugs are described in more detail below. Following this information are brief descriptions of drugs that have been used to treat fibromyalgia but are not directly approved for use in this manner. I do not explicitly endorse any drug described in this Chapter. Rather, I present this information for your consideration. You and your physician are the only two people qualified to determine what is best for you and your situation. Some drugs may need a few weeks to be effective, and then they must be taken daily for maintenance. Other drugs work immediately, but work for several hours, necessitating another drug—

and perhaps different drug—at a later time. For example, one compound may decrease your pain and fatigue and increase alertness, which would be better suited for daytime. Then, a drug that eases pain and is mildly sedating would be better for evening.

Please keep in mind that all drugs, in sufficient amounts, can have toxic or unwanted effects, which may be more intolerable than the symptoms of fibromyalgia. Also, the choice to abstain from drug therapy is always a valid decision, and it may be the best decision for many people. Please see Chapter 5 for non-drug concepts to manage fibromyalgia. Perhaps these ideas are more suitable for you, or perhaps a combination of both drug and non-drug strategies will be the best solution for your symptoms. In this chapter, prescription medications are noted with a symbol: ℞

❖ Milnacipran ℞

Milnacipran (brand name: Savella) is the newest drug approved by the FDA for fibromyalgia.[233-235] Approved for use in the US in 2009, milnacipran has been used for more than a decade in other countries such as Austria as an antidepressant. Milnacipran is a serotonin-norepinephrine re-uptake inhibitor that balances the ratios of the neurotransmitters in the nerve to improve the symptoms of depression. Scientists speculate that inhibition of norepinephrine contributes to the pain relief for people with fibromyalgia.

Something to consider when trying drugs initially indicated for depression and related syndromes to treat fibromyalgia is the time needed to achieve the full effects of the medication. For treatment of depression, 3 or 4 weeks are often required for symptoms to improve. Likewise, some time may be needed for the chronic pain of fibromyalgia to subside, and then daily maintenance may be the key to keeping symptoms under complete control. Side effects of milnacipran include nausea and difficulty urinating.

❖ Duloxetine ℞

Duloxetine (brand name: Cymbalta) is a medication indicated for depression, and in clinical studies it was promising for reducing pain in people with fibromyalgia.[227, 236, 237] Duloxetine is a selective serotonin and norepinephrine re-uptake inhibitor. This means that the drug prolongs the effects of neurotransmitters by blocking the neurotransmitter from being reabsorbed or taken back up after it has been released into the space between the nerves, the synapse. Therefore, the neurotransmitter can send signals for a greater duration. This type of re-uptake blockade is thought to be useful in controlling symptoms of depression, a disorder for which some neurotransmitters are thought to be too short-lived.[238, 239]

People who reported pain relief from duloxetine also commented that this drug produced a few adverse effects such as nausea, dry mouth, constipation, sleepiness, and agitation. Some of these side effects were severe enough to cause patients to discontinue the drug, but this occurred in a small number of individuals. If duloxetine seems to be a good idea for you, consult with a physician to learn whether any additional medications you take could interact with duloxetine. For example, duloxetine may produce adverse effects in people who are also taking monoamine oxidase inhibitors, which are another type of antidepressant. Also, glaucoma and liver problems are a concern for people taking duloxetine.

❖ Pregabalin ℞

Pregabalin (brand name: Lyrica) has been shown to be effective for people with fibromyalgia.[230, 231] Pregabalin is not a new drug, but use of this drug for fibromyalgia is considered a new drug *indication* or a new use. Previous indications for pregabalin include pain relief for diabetic neuropathy, which is a painful sensation felt in the extremities of people who have severe diabetes. Also, pregabalin has been used to control the pain of herpes lesions, referred to as post-herpetic neuralgia. Pregabalin has anti-seizure activity. Thus, anyone currently taking anti-seizure medication should consult with a physician to ensure the safety of adding a similar drug to their daily regimen.

Pregabalin acts at the alpha-2 adrenergic receptor, which was described earlier in relation to Reynaud's Syndrome. By acting on these receptors, which are tiny docking stations for drugs and other compounds, pregabalin reduces anxiety and reduces the body's response to pain. Studies with pregabalin suggest that it is well tolerated in most individuals and that it has few side effects.[230]

Off-Label Drugs Used in Fibromyalgia

The FDA approves prescription drugs for specific uses based on compelling scientific and clinical evidence. Thus, the FDA does not explicitly endorse indications or uses for prescription drugs that have not been specifically tested in that way. Instead, physicians may legally prescribe any drug on the market for a use that they determine is appropriate. This allows clinicians to be more innovative in their practices by trying new medications that might be beneficial. Also, off-label usage permits treatment flexibility for patients who do not respond to first-choice medications but who might respond to anther drug type. This type of prescribing for non-specifically approved uses is called off-label prescribing, which literally is the prescribing of a medication in a manner different from that approved by the FDA. Because strong scientific and clinical evidence for off-label uses is usually not available or does not yet exist, an off-label use for one person may not be suitable for another. Moreover, physicians may disagree with one another about the merits of an off-label use, and they have the right to refuse to prescribe a certain drug.

On the other hand, if sufficient experience with an off-label drug can be documented, a clinical practice guideline may emerge in which a drug can be recommended for use in an additional way, such as aspirin being used to decrease the risk of stroke. Initially, aspirin was used for pain relief, but when evidence was documented that aspirin could be very beneficial for stroke prevention in doses that were not associated with side effects, physicians endorsed this new indication. Now, aspirin is recommended to decrease the risk of a blood clot that could lead to a stroke.

When such safety and effectiveness can be demonstrated, and no additional risk is documented, a drug manufacturer may apply for a new drug indication by submitting a supplemental new drug application to the FDA. Then, the FDA may decide that the drug can be re-labeled to include this new use. Similarly, off-label use of drugs to treat fibromyalgia can be a good idea if the drug proves effective and safe, but use of off-label drugs can be controversial in that insurance agencies may not wish to pay for a drug that has not been approved for that specific condition. In fact, experimental therapeutics are often denied coverage by insurance agencies. Thus, if insurance coverage for medication is important to you, ask your health care provider what measures you can take, if any, to get insurance coverage for your treatment.

The drugs described below are considered off-label drugs for the treatment of fibromyalgia. Although some practice guidelines suggest that several of them are appropriate first-choice therapy for people with fibromyalgia, off-label drugs, like any drug, may not be helpful to you. Some may be harmful for you, or your physician may not agree to prescribe them for you. I do not endorse any drug listed below. I merely describe each based on the reports in the scientific literature, and I leave this important decision to you and your physician.

❖ Olanzapine ℞

Olanzapine [brand name: Zyprexa] is originally approved for the treatment of schizophrenia and bipolar disorder, two severe and difficult to treat mental disorders. How the drug works in people with fibromyalgia is not clear at this time, but scientists know that the drug blocks the neurotransmitters dopamine and serotonin. This action is different from blocking re-uptake of neurotransmitters; the neurotransmitters themselves are inhibited from acting within the synapse. Some patients with fibromyalgia have reported a decrease in their pain symptoms when taking olanzapine.[65, 229, 240, 241] Interestingly, people given olanzapine to relieve fibromyalgia-related pain reported that their pain and low tolerance for activity returned when the drug was discontinued, and that their pain decreased again when the drug was re-introduced. This would suggest that the drug is effective, and that the drug's effects are short-lived, disappearing when the medication is withdrawn. Thus, to remain pain-free, people may require a daily dose of olanzapine.

Olanzapine, like many other similar medications prescribed for mental disorders frequently have side effects that target motor functions. For example, some drugs in this class cause irreversible tremors that are similar to Tardive Dyskinesia, a disease that causes the individual to make repeated and involuntary movements with the mouth, face, upper body, or extremities. Such olanzapine side effects may affect people indiscriminately : some patients experience them when others do not.[65, 240, 241] Other side effects associated with olanzapine include hyperglycemia which could complicate pre-existing diabetes, and adverse cardiac events such as stroke.

❖ Gabapentin ℞

Gabapentin (brand name: Neurontin) is an anticonvulsant or anti-seizure medication that acts on the brain to stabilize signals. Some people with fibromyalgia, who do not take the drug for seizures, have reported a decrease in their pain symptoms with this drug.[227, 242, 243] Although gabapentin is relatively safe, some precautions must be taken. Gabapentin can cause drowsiness in some people, and anyone who experiences excessive fatigue, weakness, incoordination or tremor should consult a physician about these side effects.

Antacids taken along with gabapentin might reduce the amount of gabapentin available in the body. Also, certain drugs that reduce the production of stomach acid, specifically cimetidine (brand name: Tagamet) will reduce the ability of the kidneys to remove gabapentin from the body. Gabapentin is not recommended for pregnant women, and the safety of this drug for children under the age of 12 years is not known. Common side effects of this drug are high blood pressure, coughing, sore throat, runny nose, back pain, and arthritis-like pain, among other symptoms.

❖ Tramadol ℞

Tramadol (brand name Ultram), is an analgesic or pain reliever that has two actions in the body. First, it binds to opioid receptors, which are sites where narcotics bind in the body to relieve pain and alter the perception of pain. Also, tramadol inhibits the re-uptake of serotonin and norepinephrine. In fibromyalgia studies, tramadol was effective in relieving pain.[244, 245]

Tramadol is not a scheduled drug, and it is not considered to have addictive potential, which is important because many drugs that reduce pain by binding to opioid receptors can be habit-forming and can lead to drug abuse in susceptible individuals.[246] Common side effects of tramadol are flushing, confusion, sleepiness, nausea, diarrhea, stomach pain, vomiting, inability to void urine, increased protein and creatinine (a normal breakdown product of muscle protein) in the urine. Tramadol should not be taken with alcohol or with narcotic) or with drugs used to treat mental illness. Taking tramadol with monoamine oxidase inhibitor antidepressants may increase the risk of seizures. Tramadol is not recommended for pregnant women or children younger than 16 years-of-age.

❖ Carisoprodol ℞

Carisoprodol [brand name: Soma] is a skeletal muscle relaxant that does not directly relax muscles but works indirectly by acting at the level of the brain and the spine. For some people, this drug can be helpful for easing the pain fibromyalgia.[247, 248] Carisoprodol is normally recommended for pain due to muscle strain or muscle spasm, and the drug's anxiety-reducing and mild sedative effects are thought to augment or support its muscle relaxing effects.

Side effects of this drug include rapid heart beat, dizziness when standing due to a rapid drop in blood pressure, flushing, dizziness, sleepiness, tremor, irritability, headache, inability to sleep, nausea, vomiting, stomach pain, and rarely, rash, asthma, weakness, and allergy-related shock. Carisoprodol should not be taken with alcohol or other sedating drugs. This drug has not been fully evaluated in pregnant women, and carisoprodol has not been thoroughly tested in children under 12 years-of-age.

❖ Botulinum Toxin ℞

Botulinum toxin type A [brand name: Botox] is a neurotoxin isolated from the bacterium *Clostridium botulinum*. This compound is widely used in clinical settings to address painful muscle spasms by paralyzing the specific muscle and in dermatology and plastic surgery for paralyzing facial muscles that contribute to wrinkling and to reduce sweating by paralyzing sweat-producing structures under the arm and in the groin. Other various applications for Botulinum toxin have been reported.

Off-label use of Botulinum toxin for pain management in fibromyalgia is being investigated because Botulinum toxin injection at certain sites can stop pain-signal transmission.[249-253] In studies, Botulinum toxin was not found to be helpful for controlling the pain of fibromyalgia, and this failure could be attributed to the site of injection, the dosage, and the technique for administering the drug.[254, 255] Overall, more studies are warranted to completely rule out Botulinum toxin as a therapy for fibromyalgia pain. Botulinum toxin can have side effects, but these are not usually related to overdose. In the event of overdose, an anti-toxin (toxin reversal agent) is available. Instead, unwanted side effects from Botulinum toxin include hypersensitivities, facial sagging or drooping, and aggravation of pre-existing neuromuscular disorders.

❖ Amitriptyline ℞

Antidepressants are popular treatments for fibromyalgia, and amitriptyline (brand name: Elavil) is the most studied of the tricyclic class of antidepressants. Tricyclics are named for the 3-ring chemical structure they have in common. Amitriptyline benefits a significant population of those with fibromyalgia by increasing the amount of serotonin and norepinephrine in the central nervous system, which are neurotransmitters that produce a sense of well-being.[256-259] Interestingly, only short-term use of amitriptyline has been shown to be effective, and the drug does not appear to be helpful in long-term therapy.[256, 258, 260]

Amitriptyline can produce unwanted side effects such as cardiovascular episodes including myocardial infarction, stroke, heart block, and hypertension. Seizures can occur in certain individuals, and some people may experience rashes, tremors, restlessness, and dry mouth. For a few people, the side effects of the drugs may be worse than the actual fibromyalgia symptoms, and the drug must be discontinued.

❖ Cyclobenzaprine ℞

Cyclobenzaprine (brand name: Flexeril) is structurally similar to amitriptyline but it has a different chemical activity: it is a skeletal muscle relaxant.[261, 262] Skeletal muscle relaxants reduce muscle spasms by reducing muscle activity signals, and it is recommended for painful muscle conditions. Like amitriptyline, cyclobenzaprine is effective for short-term use but has not yet been evaluated for continual use over long periods of time.[260, 263] Cyclobenzaprine has been used in small studies with children with fibromyalgia, and positive results were reported.[264]

Cyclobenzaprine should be taken with food to reduce gastrointestinal irritation, and it should not be taken by anyone with certain types of glaucoma or liver disease. Cyclobenzaprine also should not be taken by anyone also taking certain antidepressants (monoamine oxidase inhibitors) or drugs that block the neurotransmitter acetylcholine. Acetylcholine-blocking drugs are used to treat gastrointestinal disorders such as diverticulitis, or other conditions like inflammation of the prostate. Other side effects reported for cyclobenzaprine include abdominal pain, acid reflux, constipation, and nausea.

❖ Venlafaxine ℞

Venlafaxine (brand name: Effexor) is prescribed for major depression. The drug strongly prevents re-uptake of the neurotransmitters serotonin and norepinephrine and weakly prevents dopamine re-uptake. This means that neurotransmitters stay active longer in the nerve cells. Because serotonin and norepinephrine have been reported to be low in people with fibromyalgia, this drug may improve symptoms in some people. Side effects form venlafaxine are mild and include sweating, nausea, dizziness, and tremor. In some people, venlafaxine can increase blood pressure, which is problematic for people with existing hypertension. Also, this medication should be used with caution in the elderly who may be overly sensitive to the effects.

❖ Fluoxetine ℞

Fluoxetine (brand name: Prozac) has been shown to be effective in people with fibromyalgia. This popular drug is a common drug prescribed for depression and obsessive-compulsive disorder that selectively blocks the uptake of serotonin once it is released from the nerve cell.[265-268] Like venlafaxine (discussed above), these drugs may help some people with the pain of fibromyalgia. A serious side effect that is associated with fluoxetine is serotonin syndrome, a condition characterized by agitation, hallucinations, in-coordination, nausea, and vomiting. For some people, abrupt discontinuation of fluoxetine may cause irritability, dizziness, anxiety, and confusion. Fluoxetine can interact with several drugs and increase their toxicity. For example, fluoxetine can interact with carbamazepine and phenytoin (used for seizures), and other monoamine oxidase inhibitor antidepressants.

❖ Paroxetine ℞

Paroxetine (brand name: Paxil) is an antidepressant prescribed for major depressive disorder, obsessive-compulsive disorder, and other anxiety issues. Paroxetine is a selective serotonin re-uptake inhibitor, like fluoxetine and venlafaxine. Paroxetine has been shown in small studies to be helpful in reducing some symptoms of fibromyalgia but not the pain associated with fibromyalgia.[269, 270] Side effects reported for paroxetine include nausea, tremor, confusion, vomiting, and dizziness. Other adverse effects from paroxetine include confusion, rapid heart beat, and impaired concentration. Also, paroxetine can cause fatal reactions when taken with monoamine oxidase inhibitor antidepressants.

❖ Vitamin D

Vitamin D, which you can obtain from sitting in the sun or eating and drinking vitamin D supplemented foods is needed for health. Evidence is emerging that current recommendations for vitamin D are probably low, that many people have less than optimal levels of circulating vitamin D.[271, 272] Thus, additional vitamin D in the form of supplements might be beneficial to many people.[273-278] Studies to determine whether people with muscular pain had abnormally low levels of vitamin D were negative: low vitamin D does not appear to contribute to muscular pain.[279] Thus, additional vitamin D should not improve fibromyalgia symptoms.

❖ Myer's Cocktail ℞

This nutritional concoction is intravenously administered, and is suggested to help with various clinical conditions. Presently, this solution is comprised of magnesium, calcium, B vitamins, and vitamin C.[280] This preparation allegedly is useful in asthma, fatigue, upper respiratory tract infections, and fibromyalgia. The range of applications alleged for this cocktail stretch credibility at times, and there is little peer-reviewed, controlled research into the mechanisms behind how this solution is supposed to work. What is reported suggests that this preparation might have minimal risk, but the benefit is not well studied and at this time is largely anecdotal.[281, 282]

❖ Melatonin

Melatonin, which is produced by our bodies in response to our circadian rhythms that are set by sunlight, is released to produce drowsiness. Melatonin can also be taken as a supplement and is often used to help people sleep. Because of the unrefreshing sleep that accompanies fibromyalgia, melatonin was studied as a potential therapy. In a small pilot study, melatonin supplementation before bedtime was found to improve sleep in people with fibromyalgia.[283] Also, melatonin levels were measured in people with fibromyalgia and these results were compared to people who did not have fibromyalgia. There were no differences in melatonin between the two groups.[284, 285] Because of melatonin's relatively safe profile, it may be useful for improving restful sleep some people.

❖ Raloxifene ℞

Raloxifene (brand name: Evista) is a selective estrogen receptor modulator that is used to prevent osteoporosis in post-menopausal women. This means that it binds to the estrogen receptor, blocking estrogen from binding while simultaneously mimicking the effects of estrogen. Some effects of estrogen include increases in bone mineral density and decreases in total cholesterol and low-density lipid cholesterols. Raloxifene is reported to be helpful for reducing pain and fatigue in a small study of postmenopausal women with fibromyalgia.[286] More studies are needed to determine whether this drug is suitable for additional populations. Raloxifene can cause nausea, migraine, insomnia, and leg cramps in some people. Also, the safety of raloxifene has not yet been evaluated in women who are pre-menopausal.

❖ Neurotropin ℞

Neurotropin is an unusual analgesic frequently used in Japan and China. It is a polysaccharide (compound made of multiple sugar molecules) that is extracted from the skin of rabbits treated with vaccinia virus, which is closely related to the virus that causes cowpox. Neurotropin has been tested in a small study for fibromyalgia with promising results.[287, 288] Neurotropin does not inhibit the body's ability to produce prostaglandins, which means that the drug is not effective for inflammation-based pain that is due to prostaglandins. This also means that the drug does not cause stomach irritation commonly attributed to agents that block prostaglandins. Nevertheless, additional studies with more research subjects are necessary to confirm that this drug is safe and beneficial for people with fibromyalgia.

❖ Non-steroidal Anti-inflammatory Drugs

Various forms of non-steroidal anti-inflammatory drugs such as acetaminophen, ibuprofen, and naproxen have been tried in fibromyalgia, but none were found to be particularly helpful. Because fibromyalgia is not an inflammatory condition, it would be reasonable to conclude that these drugs would have little or no effect in most people. Still, use of these agents in people with fibromyalgia is common medical practice.[289]

❖ Narcotic Drugs ℞

Narcotics are not presented in this Chapter as a real or practical solutions for fibromyalgia. This class of drugs is not particularly useful in managing the daily pain of fibromyalgia. Narcotics act on the brain to change the way we perceive pain in addition to reducing the sensation of certain types of pain. In some people, narcotics may produce a feeling of wellbeing and give them the sensation that their pain is decreased. For others, nausea and profound sedation or sleepiness may be experienced with prescribed doses of narcotics, and pain relief may be variable. Narcotics can also be habit-forming or addictive.[290-292] Some physicians advocate prescribing narcotics to people in chronic pain, even in the face of an addiction, but the risks associated with this practice are under debate, and patient monitoring is essential.[290, 292]

Also, narcotics can be dangerous when combined with alcohol. For some people, the activities of daily living such as driving a car or working in the yard can be dangerous because narcotics can impair judgment in susceptible persons, although the literature suggests that people under the influence of narcotics are not significantly different from non-medicated persons when operating a motor vehicle or engaging in similar activities. Thus, a person can become acclimated to—or accustomed to the effects of—narcotics.

Also, physicians are reluctant to prescribe narcotics in an open-ended fashion for pain that is not related to something serious such as post-surgical pain or pain related to a major disease such as cancer. The US Drug Enforcement Agency monitors narcotic prescriptions, and physicians who frequently prescribe these types of medications without fully documenting the need for such prescriptions can come under scrutiny or worse, can lose their prescribing rights and privileges.[293] Often, patients do not realize the seriousness associated with frequent narcotic prescribing when they demand these drugs from their health care provider. Thus, because narcotics simply do not target the reason behind fibromyalgia pain and they can increase the sensation of sedation or fatigue, these drugs are simply not suitable for managing fibromyalgia day to day.

❖ Injectable Drugs ℞

Injectable medications—drugs that can be administered intravenously (into the vein), intramuscularly (into the muscle), or subcutaneously (under the skin)—have been explored for people with fibromyalgia.[294] Both growth hormone and local anesthetics have been administered, with various outcomes. Some people responded to the injections, and others did not respond at all.[294] Growth hormone, which tells the body to produce insulin-like growth factor (IGF), was thought to be useful for people with fibromyalgia who had low levels of IGF. Of the 26 studies conducted, only three were suggestive of some benefit of injecting growth hormone to raise IGF.

Intravenous administration of ketamine or lidocaine was reported to reduce pain in tested groups.[295, 296] Ketamine is labeled for general anesthesia and lidocaine is both an anti-arrhythmic drug for the heart as well as a local anesthetic. Ketamine has been given orally to participants of one study and it was reported to reduce chronic pain.[297] Ketamine must be cautiously used by people with psychiatric disorders such as schizophrenia and acute psychoses. Also, people with hypertension (elevated blood pressure) may not be able to tolerate this compound.

Lidocaine can be dangerous for people who have hypersensitivity to local anesthetics similar to lidocaine, and lidocaine toxicity can occur with repeated administrations of this drug. Persons also taking medication for heart conditions should use caution when considering lidocaine for fibromyalgia relief.

Drug Development and Research

We are enjoying unprecedented growth in drug research and therapeutic availability as new drugs come to market, older drugs become accessible over the counter and without a prescription, and as we find new uses for existing compounds. For most symptoms or illness, excellent drugs or therapies are usually available to treat or manage the condition. This is not the case for fibromyalgia, despite the 60 years of research into the clinical question of what causes the disorder and the attempts to treat multiple aspects of this complex disease.

Thus, as of 2009, there are only three approved drugs indicated for fibromyalgia. This is partly because identifying a true target for fibromyalgia therapy is difficult. For example, scientists who develop the drug must decide if the drug should target the pain of fibromyalgia, or whether the drug should alleviate the actual problem that is causing the pain, which could be the over-sensitized nervous system. Because research into why the pain occurs is just expanding, meaningful therapies are scarce. Also, the time required to develop, test, and market a drug is lengthy and expensive.

Surprisingly, fewer than a quarter (25%) of all drugs and therapeutics tested for drug development eventually come out at the end of the drug discovery process as useful products. Drug development is typically a 7–8-year process and from the early 1960s to 1999, fewer than 20 new drugs a year were approved for marketing.[298, 299] So, a new drug for fibromyalgia is certainly fortuitous.

❖ Models Used in Drug Development

When scientists want to understand how a disease is caused or how it can be treated or cured, they turn to systems or models that mimic the disease state in humans. Animals are commonly used in laboratories for this purpose, and they are referred to as *experimental models*. Although animal studies may not perfectly predict all aspects of a particular illness, many animals are excellent representatives for humans. For example, the hearts of turkeys can mimic pathological changes in some diseased human hearts, the epidermis of the swine and the a particular type of guinea pig is a good tool for studying human skin; some breeds of mice are useful in studying the kidney, and the dog is an excellent model for the aging human brain.[300-305]

The animal model for fibromyalgia is a rat and mouse model of chronic pain because scientists have found that these animals most closely approximate what people experience when subjected to painful stimuli.[306, 307] Fibromyalgia is largely diagnosed through the actual *communication* of perceived pain, and animals cannot speak, so scientists have devised methods for accurately measuring what the animal is "feeling" but cannot express. For example, scientists can apply a cold substance to the paws of the animals, which is a painful—but not harmful—stimuli for the rodents. Then, they can measure their response to the cold by measuring circulating neurotransmitters and then test whether therapies change the neurotransmitter concentration.[308 309]

Sometimes, people respond to news about animal studies in very emotional ways. Frequently, the public experiences a surge in interest in animal studies, and several fringe groups seek to disrupt experimental animal research. For example, some animal rights groups will break in to laboratories and release animals from cages, causing thousands of dollars in damage and destruction. This is an unfortunate practice because it discourages scientists from sharing animal experimental research and it ultimately delays the creation and dissemination of new knowledge.[310-312]

The public should understand that no scientist would undertake animal experimentation without a sound rationale for the experimentation and ethical justification for the use of that particular animal.[313, 314] Also, the animal research that is performed in the US (and likely other countries) is overseen by a review panel which has rigorous guidelines which all scientists follow or risk the loss of their research funding, or worse, loss of their job. All scientists performing research under these guidelines strive to minimize the total number of animals used in any experiment and recognize the need to reduce or eliminate the unnecessary pain and distress that may be experienced by these animas in research.

❖ Clinical Trials

When drugs are studied in humans in a formal fashion, they are referred to as clinical trials. In fact, before any drug is sold to the public, it has been investigated under a clinical trial, and most drugs proceed through the trials in phases. Phase I trials involved only a small number of healthy people who volunteer to participate in the research. The purpose of a phase I trials is to learn what effects an investigational compound has in human subjects such as how it travels through the body, whether it is changed when passing through the body, and how it leaves the body. This information tells the researchers about the safety and tolerability of the new drug because volunteers are carefully monitored for side effects.

Phase II clinical studies are similar to Phase I studies but they are conducted in people who have a specific disease or condition that the drug was designed to treat. So, in addition to evaluating side effects and safety, the researchers are also measuring how well the drug works for that condition, or the efficacy of the compound. Participants in Phase II trials are similar with respect to their disease or condition and they are given various doses of the compound. The effects are then compared to find the safest dosing regimen. Other accepted treatments for that disease may also be compared to the drug under investigation to determine if one is better.

In Phase III trials, the safety, efficacy, and dosage are again measured but in much larger populations than Phase II or I trials. Prescribing information is gained from these trials and this information is submitted to regulatory agencies for consideration and approval. After approval, Phase IV trials or post-market surveillance trials are conducted to provide even more comprehensive information about the safety and efficacy of the drug. Usually, during Phase IV, sufficient people are given the drug such that odd reactions may be observed for the first time. This does not mean that the drug was or is unsafe, it simply means that an individual had an unusual response, which can be expected if enough people are given a drug...eventually at least one person will have an interesting reaction. This is simply the cost we bear of being genetically unique individuals with different susceptibilities.

Evaluation of Scientific Information

At this time, only 3 drugs are indicated (approved for use) for fibromyalgia. The remainder of the drugs described in this book are legitimate compounds with other indications, but they also have been reported to be useful in people with fibromyalgia. When evaluating studies that report positive effects for a drug not initially indicated for fibromyalgia, you should keep a few facts in mind. First, note the number of people studied. If only 10 people were evaluated in the drug study, you might conclude that this population was too small to truly measure the drug's effects. Large sample sizes increase the likelihood of finding meaningful results.

Also, you should look for the inclusion of study subjects who did not receive the drug under investigation. This means that the study was controlled: some participants received the study drug and others received a *placebo* or *control*, which is a "dummy" drug, "sugar pill", or a drug-like product that lacks the active ingredient being tested. Controls are necessary in drug research to accurately measure the effects of the drug. Ideally, in a well-controlled study with an appropriate drug, the population that received the real drug improved, and the control population that received the placebo or sugar pill did not improve.

Randomization is another sign of a good study design. This means that study participants are assigned to receive the study drug or the placebo in an unplanned manner—in a random way. Randomization is thought to prevent bias in results that can skew the data in the wrong direction. Also, blinded studies are better than open studies. In open studies, everyone knows whether the study participant received the study drug or the placebo. This can greatly affect the outcome of the study because people who get the real drug may report a greater benefit, whether they really benefitted more or not. A single-blind study means that the study participant does not know for sure if he received the study drug or the placebo until the study is over and the results are tabulated. Having a double blind investigation means that both the researcher and the study participant are unaware of which drug is assigned. Double blind studies often produce more reliable data than single blind studies.

Other hallmarks of a well-executed study include comparisons of study subjects that were matched for age, health, and gender. Obviously comparing elderly subjects who took the drug with children who received the placebo does not make sense. The differences between the groups might be explained by the drug or the age or health of the individuals in the group. Likewise, for some drug studies, men should be compared to other age-matched men, and women should be compared with age-matched women because gender differences in drug response have been known to occur. Overall, when evaluating clinical studies for new medications or new uses for old medications, look for studies that are well-planned and appropriately conducted to draw the best conclusions about whether a drug treatment is effective.

❖ The Placebo Effect

In clinical trials, participants sometimes declare that they receive a benefit from the placebo. This phenomenon is referred to as a *placebo effect*. The concept of a placebo effect is unique because—quite literally—a placebo should have *no* effect. Some people believe that the perception of a benefit from a placebo is due to an individual's lack of education or intellect, or worse, the gullibility of the person. This is not true. Everyone is susceptible to a placebo effect because our brains cannot help but anticipate a benefit from simply taking a drug.

When scientists report that study participants experience a placebo effect that mimics the real drug effects, the treatment is not concluded to be ineffective. Rather, the treatment is considered to be not different than placebo.[315-317] Interestingly, the placebo effect—in its purest form—can be beneficial to those with fibromyalgia. If a person with fibromyalgia is told that his daily walks with the dog are exercise, and that this exercise is good for him, he is more likely to feel good about the dog walking. The activity becomes a form of self-care, providing a sense of control and accomplishment. This type of positive mind-set was observed in hotel housekeepers who were told that their work was the equivalent of exercise. After being told this, the housekeeping staff believed that they were exercising more, and their weight, blood pressure, and body fat improved significantly.[318]

When discussing drug therapy, it is important to consider that one drug may help one person but be useless for another. What your friend may describe about a drug may differ from how it works with your body. Thus, never take a drug solely on the advice of a friend. Scientists and physicians refer to this type of information as *anecdotal*. An anecdote is similar to a personal tale or a story, and it is less reliable than an evidence-based fact. The best drug data are derived from proper drug studies in which many data sets are compared, sifted, and statistically analyzed to produce reliable conclusions. Such rigor makes drug study data more powerful and relevant than Aunt Ruth's opinion about a medication. Also, simply hearing *many* anecdotes about a drug still does not mean that you have information that rises to the level of valid or relevant data. Thus, regard with care the information provided by well-meaning friends and family, and always get proper medical advice before starting a drug or regimen.

Chapter Summary

- ❖ Three drugs are approved for fibromyalgia: milnacipran (Savella), pregabalin (Lyrica), and duloxetine (Cymbalta).
- ❖ Other off-label drugs have been used with some success for people with fibromyalgia: olanzapine, gabapentin, tramadol, carisoprodol amitriptyline cyclobenzaprine, venlafaxine, fluoxetine, paroxetine, and others.
- ❖ Drug research is ongoing to find new therapies for fibromyalgia.
- ❖ Animal models of chronic pain syndromes are helpful in the investigation of new therapies.
- ❖ Humans can participate in research into new therapies by joining clinical trials for new drugs.
- ❖ The best drug studies are randomized, double-blind designs that test a control or non-drug compound with the study drug in sufficient numbers of people.

CHAPTER 5—NON-DRUG TREATMENTS FOR FIBROMYALGIA

Some people do not prefer to treat themselves with drugs because of previous drug intolerances, the cost of using drugs, or current pre-existing conditions which complicate finding a suitable drug that will not interfere with other health conditions or treatments. Truly, many drugs do not work well for all people with fibromyalgia, and some do not work at all. Also, problems with insurance or the cost of therapies presents a real and significant burden for many; often physicians are unaware of the costs of therapies that they prescribe.[319] Thus, drugs to treat fibromyalgia may not be accessible for some people.

Thus, nonpharmacological approaches may be a first choice for many. Also, non-pharmacological or non-drug therapies are wonderful adjuncts or additional techniques for increasing wellness and decreasing pain and fatigue. The non-drug ideas presented in this Chapter are moderate-to low cost and may even be free in some areas. Also, all active and passive participation suggestions presented here are virtually risk-free, which may be appealing for many people who are willing to try something new. Each active-participation option can be modified for ability and tolerance to the specific activity.

Active Participation Treatments

❖ Aquatic Therapy

Several non-pharmacologic or drug-free approaches to treating fibromyalgia are gaining popularity and scientific studies indicate that many are effective. For example, aquatic therapy—perhaps in the form of water aerobics, offered by health clubs and community centers—has been shown to be very good for fibromyalgia. In one study, women with fibromyalgia participated in aquatic exercise in a warm pool of waist-high water.[320, 321] These women experienced pain relief, increased quality of life, and increased muscle strength in their lower limbs. In other studies with aquatic exercise programs, similar results were reported.[322] These benefits obtained from exercising in a pool were sustained over time, too.[321]

Obviously, with water-based exercises, two variables are interacting—the warm water, and the aerobic activity of the participant. Interestingly, warm water treatment, like that enjoyed in a spa bath or hot tub, without specific aerobic exercise has been shown to be effective in improving mood, sleep quality, and fatigue. Interestingly, when statistics were applied to compare whether people who enjoyed spa baths for their fibromyalgia experienced less benefit than those who aerobically exercised in warm water, the conclusion from the statistical analysis was that both groups fared equally well.[323, 324] Clearly, this is excellent news for people with severe and incapacitating fibromyalgia who need to start with more passive activities and progress to more vigorous exercises.

❖ Yoga

Yoga is originally an Indian form of exercise, of which there are several forms. The term *yoga* loosely can be translated from the Sanskrit to mean *to control* or *to unite*. Variations of yoga-like practices such as meditation, relaxation, and breathing techniques are also good starting points for coping with fibromyalgia, although rigorous have not concluded that there is an absolute benefit at this time.[325-327] Yogic postures, called *asanas*, can be specifically applied to address the painful areas.

For example, poses that stretch the hamstrings and lower back may alleviate tenderness for people who report particular pain in that area. Because yoga poses or postures can be grouped according to the area of the body they target, exercises can be chosen to directly address what you need on any day. Because yoga asanas are named in the language of the practice, Sanskrit, the asanas listed below are accompanied by their common English translation. In some yoga practices, the common name may be a little different, but the Sanskrit name should be the same.

Teaching the how-to of yoga poses is beyond the scope of this book. However, if you already practice yoga, you can add these asanas to your routine. If you have never practiced yoga and you want to try a few poses, you can take this list to any yoga studio or location where yoga classes are offered [YMCA, YWCA, community center, etc.] and ask the *yogi* [yoga teacher] how to perform the asanas. Most yogis are very helpful and would be delighted to show you some poses or even to add some of your requested poses to the class you attend. Also, most yogis should be able to suggest a variation for each pose that best suits your flexibility. The table below presents some yoga asanas that are grouped according to their target areas. This list is not exhaustive but it is a good starting point.

If you have never tried yoga, this table may present some interesting information for experimenting. You may even choose a few poses to use as stretches as you need them. Thus, the information can be used many ways.

TABLE 1 YOGA POSES TARGETED TO SPECIFIC AREAS	Targeted Area						
Yoga Asana/Pose Sanskrit name (English common name)	Hands/fingers	Buttocks	Hamstrings	Neck	Lower back	Upper back	Thighs
Adho Mukha Svanasana (Downward-Facing Dog)	■		■		■	■	
Agnistambhasana (Fire Log Pose)		■					
Ananda Balasana (Happy Baby Pose)		■	■				
Anantasana (Side-Reclining Leg Lift)			■				
Anjali Mudra (Salutation Seal)	■						
Anjaneyasana (Low Lunge)					■		
Ardha Bhekasana (Half Frog Pose)		■					■
Ardha Chandrasana (Half Moon Pose)					■		
Ardha Matsyendrasana (Half Lord of the Fishes Pose)					■	■	
Ardha Uttanasana (Standing Half Forward Bend)			■				
Baddha Konasana (Bound Angle Pose)			■				
Bakasana (Crane Pose)	■						■
Bharadvajasana I (Bharadvaja's Twist)						■	
Bhujangasana (Cobra Pose)	■				■		
Bitilasana (Cow Pose)				■			
ButtocksPadangusthasana (Big Toe Pose)		■					
Chaturanga Dandasana (Four-Limbed Staff Pose)	■						
Dandasana (Staff Pose)			■	■			
Dhanurasana (Bow Pose)					■	■	
Dolphin Plank Pose					■		
Dolphin Pose					■	■	
Dwi Pada Viparita Dandasana (Upward Facing Two-Foot Staff Pose)		■					
Eka Pada Koundiyanasana I (Pose Dedicated to the Sage Koundinya I)					■		
Eka Pada Koundiyanasana II (Pose Dedicated					■		

TABLE 1 YOGA POSES TARGETED TO SPECIFIC AREAS

Yoga Asana/Pose Sanskrit name (English common name)	Hands/fingers	Buttocks	Hamstrings	Neck	Lower back	Upper back	Thighs
to the Sage Koundinya II)					■	■	
Eka Pada Rajakapotasana (One-Legged King Pigeon Pose)							■
Eka Pada Rajakapotasana II (One-Legged King Pigeon Pose II)				■			
Garudasana (Eagle Pose)							
Gomukhasana (Cow Face Pose)							
Hanumanasana (Monkey Pose)			■				
High Lunge			■				
Janu Sirsasana (Head-to-Knee Forward Bend)			■				
Krounchasana (Heron Pose)							■
Malasana (Garland Pose)					■		
Marichyasana I (Pose Dedicated to the Sage Marichi, I)			■				
Marichyasana III (Marichi's Pose)					■		
Marjaryasana (Cat Pose)				■	■		
Matsyasana (Fish Pose)				■		■	
Mayurasana (Peacock Pose)		■					■
Natarajasana (Lord of the Dance Pose)							
Padangusthasana (Big Toe Pose)			■				
Parighasana (Gate Pose)							
Parivrtta Janu Sirsasana (Revolved Head-to-Knee Pose)			■				
Parsva Bakasana (Side Crane Pose)					■		
Parsvottanasana (Intense Side Stretch Pose)			■				
Pasasana (Noose Pose)							■
Paschimottanasana (Seated Forward Bend)			■			■	
Plank Pose	■						
Prasarita Padottanasana (Wide-Legged Forward Bend)			■				
Purvottanasana (Upward Plank Pose)	■			■			■
Salamba Sarvangasana (Supported Shoulderstand)		■			■	■	
Salamba Sirsasana (Supported Headstand)		■	■		■		
Salambhasana (Locust Pose)		■	■		■		
Setu Bandha Sarvangasana (Bridge Pose)							
Simhasana (Lion Pose)	■						

TABLE 1 YOGA POSES TARGETED TO SPECIFIC AREAS

Yoga Asana/Pose Sanskrit name (English common name)	Hands/fingers	Buttocks	Hamstrings	Neck	Lower back	Upper back	Thighs
Sphinx Pose		▪		▪	▪		
Sukhasana (Easy Pose)					▪		
Supta Padangusthasana (Reclining Big Toe Pose)			▪				▪
Supta Virasana (Reclining Hero Pose)					▪		▪
Tadasana (Mountain Pose)		▪					▪
Tittibhasana (Firefly Pose)			▪				
Triangle Pose					▪		
Upavistha Konasana (Wide-Angle Seated Forward Bend)			▪				▪
Urdhva Dhanurasana (Upward Bow or Wheel Pose)	▪	▪					
Urdhva Mukha Svanasana (Upward-Facing Dog)					▪		▪
Urdhva Prasarita Eka Padasana (Standing Split)			▪				
Urdhva Prasarita Eka Padasana (Standing Split)							▪
Ustrasana (Camel Pose)					▪		
Utkatasana (Chair Pose)							▪
Uttana Shishosana (Extended Puppy Pose)						▪	
Uttanasana (Standing Forward Bend)			▪				
Utthita Hasta Padangustasana (Extended Hand-To-Big-Toe Pose)	▪		▪				
Utthita Trikonasana (Extended Triangle Pose)		▪					
Vasisthasana (Side Plank Pose)		▪					
Viparita Karani (Legs-Up-the-Wall Pose)			▪				
Virabhadrasana I (Warrior I Pose)					▪		
Virabhadrasana II (Warrior II Pose)						▪	
Virabhadrasana III (Warrior III Pose)			▪				
Virasana (Hero Pose)							▪
Vrksasana (Tree Pose)						▪	

❖ Tai Chi and Other Eastern Practices

Tai Chi, an ancient Chinese exercise that combines physical exercise with mind and body therapy, and Qi Gong, which is practiced in China as a way to maintain health by focusing on the body's energy, have been shown to be somewhat beneficial in small studies.[326, 328-330] These practices pose little or no risk to the individual, and they might be interesting for adventurous types. The concentration on breathing and the slow, controlled motions can help people with fibromyalgia to relax, which may help in managing pain and fatigue. Some community centers and recreation facilities offer classes for these practices, so you only have to call and inquire.

❖ Meditation

Meditation, which originated in the East, is gaining acceptance in Western cultures. Meditation calls for an individual to focus on a point of reference—perhaps a distant area of a wall or a nature scene outside the window—and to relax while controlling the breath. Meditation can be helpful to people with fibromyalgia, but controlled studies to explain its benefits are lacking.[326] Also, *mindfulness*, which is simply a conscious state of being aware and present in the moment, can be helpful for people dealing with multiple and overwhelming symptoms of fibromyalgia. Meditation can be incorporated into your day in many ways. Perhaps you will choose to meditate for 3 minutes at work, closing your eyes and focusing on breathing in and out. Some people take a walk outside to meditate among the trees and grass. People with excellent compartmentalization skills may be able to meditate on the drive to or from work, perhaps using a tape or CD in the car to help them relax. Some people suggest that 10 minutes of meditation before bedtime is a wonderful way to forget the day, prepare for tomorrow, and relax before sleeping.

❖ Pilates

The Pilates Method—currently referred to simply as *Pilates*—is a highly popular exercise program that dates back to the 1970's. In its present form, Pilates exercises focus on the muscles that support posture, or the core. Pilates has elements of yoga in that breath control and care of the back and spine are emphasized. In Pilates, the *core* is comprised of the abdomen, lower back, hips, and buttocks. The principle behind Pilates is that the core gives the body power and support, and a weak core is thought to be the source of injury and instability.

Pilates can be performed with the help of specific machines or devices that are designed for Pilates exercises, but more popular are Pilates exercises that are exclusively done on the floor or a mat. Numerous books and video tapes/CDs/DVDs offering instruction in Pilates exercises can be bought or checked out from the library. Also, many health clubs have certified Pilates instructors and classes for members or guests. Pilates is versatile and can be tailored to any physical ability or body type. If this exercise interests you, investigate some classes in your area. Trying exercises at home with a free video from the library or a purchased DVD may be what suits you the most. Experimenting with different types of instruction and formats will help you decide what you prefer.

❖ Aerobic Exercise

Vigorous activity is correlated with more profound pain relief in fibromyalgia. Specifically, aerobic exercise, also called cardiovascular training, is excellent for controlling or alleviating the pain and fatigue associated with fibromyalgia.[331, 332] In studies of women who were given aerobic exercise programs, participants did not adhere to the program well, which is understandable considering that fibromyalgia does not predispose many to get up and get moving.

Still, for those who did commit to a routine, the benefits were undeniable.[333-336] Exercise is an especially important consideration for people with fibromyalgia because studies show that people with fibromyalgia expend about half the calories as their normal counterparts during the day, because they instinctively choose more passive activities that will not cause fatigue.[337] Unfortunately, this tendency to avoid movement can lead to weight gain and further health complications for people with fibromyalgia.

In fact, people with fibromyalgia who developed and maintained an exercise plan of some intensity reported feeling worse if they *stopped* their exercise program.[338] This concept should be very motivating for initiating an exercise program and committing to daily movement. Researchers suggest that exercise is often overlooked in fibromyalgia treatment, so this becomes an important facet of self-management.[339] Exercising in groups improves adherence to exercise and provides a support network of others who exercise and who can motivate each another and offer accountability for those who tend to create barriers to their own exercise.[340]

A final note is that aerobic exercise need not be performed at a formal environment such as a gym or by running outside in all kinds of weather, dodging cars and unleashed dogs; rather, aerobic exercise can be anything that elevates your heart rate for about 20 to 30 uninterrupted minutes. Salsa dancing, hula-hooping, biking, hiking, or swimming can all offer aerobic activity of various intensity, so if you really love a particular activity that gets you moving, go for it!

❖ Weight Training

Lifting weights or strength training is very good for controlling fibromyalgia pain and fatigue. Also, the strength gains you acquire from consistently lifting weights is recommended for battling the normal signs of aging—muscle wasting and weight gain—and maintaining bone density, which is crucial for prolonged good health. Activities that strengthen bones are special considerations for women who lose bone density at a greater rate after menopause.[341-344]

Interestingly, adding weight training to an aerobic regimen *enhances* the effects of cardiovascular exercise. Not only are you controlling your weight by burning calories, but also you are adding shape and definition to your body by strengthening muscles.[345-347] The idea that women can become large and bulky—as men sometimes can—from weight lifting has been thoroughly debunked.[347] Women simply do not make sufficient testosterone, the hormone that assists men in creating large muscles, to form huge muscles.

Also, body builders spend hours a day lifting weights according to very prescribed regimens, and they tailor their diets to maximize their weight gains. Regular people just do not invest such time, and are often disinterested in the caloric restriction and nutrient calculus that must accompany this type of body shaping. Thus, the idea that you should not lift weights because you do not want to become large and bulky is absolutely ridiculous.[348] Weight lifting has an additional advantage for people with fibromyalgia. Lifting heavy weights to strengthen the muscles will fatigue the muscles, which is helpful at night for promoting sleep. Truly tired muscles will beckon you to lie down and sleep so that they can recover, which might improve your ability to fall and stay asleep.

The literature offers many studies to suggest that active participation in fibromyalgia management is ultimately high-benefit and low-risk. Interestingly, the barriers to increasing the quality of life in people with fibromyalgia seem to be the sufferers themselves, which is understandable. Fibromyalgia patients tend to drop out of exercise evaluations and report that exercise is stressful and difficult. More studies are warranted to find incentives for people with fibromyalgia to begin and stay with exercise because once exercise is begun in earnest and approached as a daily must-have, the positive effects are reinforcing.

Hopefully, this information about active participation in controlling symptoms of fibromyalgia will be useful and inspiring to those who currently have an exercise plan, perhaps inviting them to add some new elements to increase their pain-free moments and improve wellness. For those who have no exercise program or are initially unwilling to embark on one, perhaps this section will provide some new thoughts about interesting possibilities for fibromyalgia symptom control.

Passive Participation Treatments

❖ Acupuncture

Acupuncture has been used as a treatment for fibromyalgia.[349, 350] Acupuncture is the practice of inserting thread-like needles into the skin to relieve pain and relax the body. This practice, which has Eastern origins dating back thousands of years, is thought to stimulate the body's center of energy, referred to as *qi*. This energy has never been actually located or characterized by modern medicine or science, but it is thought to exist in the mind of the acupuncture practitioner and client, meaning that this energy is considered to be more of a concept or a virtual energy.

This virtual energy of qi is reported to flow down the body via channels called meridians, and these meridians guide the placement of the acupuncture needles. Following along the meridians, thin acupuncture needles are tapped lightly into the skin and left in place for a period of time during which the client relaxes in a dim room, perhaps on a table much like a massage table. Acupuncture is less directed at addressing a discrete biomedical or health problem, but it is used to enhance the energetic order in the body, which is thought to be the source of illness and discomfort.

The idea behind acupuncture, which is not directly supported in the peer-reviewed scientific literature, is that tapping needles into these vial energy meridians restores the harmony of the body and realigns the body's vital energy. Thus, scientific research into acupuncture has yielded conflicting findings. For example, some studies report that acupuncture is no better than no treatment at all.[351] Another study yielded results that indicated the pain associated with fibromyalgia was not significantly diminished but that the fatigue improved.[352] Yet another study revealed that people with fibromyalgia slept better after acupuncture treatments.[353, 354] Recent investigations suggest that acupuncture increases levels of neurochemicals such as serotonin and natural pain relief modulators called endorphins and related compounds, but not all studies were conducted in the same way, so questions remain.[355]

At this time, acupuncture is regarded as a *complementary alternative medicine*, much like herbal supplementation. The alternative aspect arises from the fact that these practices are not considered to be mainstream medical ideas, but they are regarded as adjuncts (complements) to traditional medical care such as physicals and prescription medication. As acupuncture, yoga, meditation, and other ideas about our mind and body become more accepted, these ideas will probably be less "alternative" than they are presently considered by medical professionals. Instead, these concepts may be viewed as essential complements to traditional Western medicine, if the scientific data show that these health regimes provide real benefit that can be replicated in many different people.

❖ Massage

Massage has origins in Eastern medicine but currently enjoys popularity all over the US. Spas that offer massage services and specifically focused massage centers are cropping up everywhere, from large cities to small rural towns. Thus, people with fibromyalgia have an excellent chance of finding massage therapy options that are both suitable for their needs and affordable. Massage is a technique of soft tissue manipulation, and studies suggest that massage is useful for alleviating pain associated with fibromyalgia.[356, 357] Also, the relaxation provided by massage may be conducive to more restful sleep, which can be beneficial. In fact, massage has been reported to benefit the muscles, tendons, ligaments, skin, joints, or other connective tissue, as well as the lymphatic system.

Specialists who perform massage are certified or licensed in massage therapy or a similar discipline, and they should have sufficient knowledge of physiology and anatomy to correctly refer to muscles and appropriately treat the body. Even so, requirements for practitioners may vary across regions. Massage methods also differ among practitioners, but most commonly, massage therapists use their hands and arms, the actions of which may be supplemented by mechanical devices that roll or heat the skin. Because massage therapy is a professional service, clients should be treated in clean and comfortable surroundings, perhaps lying on a special massage table or sitting upright in a chair.

At finer spas and locations, clients may request a male or female therapist in addition to the type or intensity of massage desired. Along with these preferences, the massage therapist will ask if there are any problems that need to be addressed or avoided. This is the perfect time for you to mention your fibromyalgia and state your wishes about the massage. A good therapist will ask *during* the massage if the pressure is too light or too heavy. Be honest, and tell the therapist exactly what you need. Prices for massage therapy may vary depending on the duration of the service. Typical therapy sessions last one-half to one hour, with longer services being more expensive. Multiple sessions may be purchased at once time at a discounted rate.

❖ Heat Therapy

An electric or microwaveable heating pad to provide dry or moist heat is an inexpensive method for relieving pain in discrete areas of the body. Most electric heating pads have fully adjustable temperature controls, and some manufacturers carry expanded heating pad sizes to cover larger areas. Many units have an automatic shut-off feature to reduce the risk of burns or fires should someone fall asleep while using the heating pad. Electric heating pads are excellent for use at home where having an electric connection is handy. Traveling with electric heating pads may prove problematic when getting through airport security and when travelling to places with unreliable or unusual electrical currents.

Non-electric heating pads are also available, and these can be heated in a microwave. Cotton (flannel, denim, etc) bags filled with field corn, flax seeds, or rice (or synthetic filler) are heated according to the instructions on the package, and the warm bag can be molded around body contours. Because these heating pads will cool over time, there is little danger of burns and virtually no danger of fire. Non-electric heating pads are useful for travel and can be heated in the morning and used in the car on the way to work. Then, the heating pad can be re-heated later in the office break room microwave and used as needed during the day. If you do not have the option of purchasing a heating pad, you can always make one with a small towel that is heated for about 1 minute in the microwave (watch for burning).

❖ Awareness and Self-Help Groups

Fibromyalgia awareness groups or self-help organizations can be life-changing experiences for those who participate. Studies show that self-help groups offer support, sympathy, and education which can have immediate and lasting effects for those who have fibromyalgia as well as for those who support or give care to people with fibromyalgia.[358, 359]

Support groups empower people with fibromyalgia to ask their physicians questions about their care, demand access to studies about their disease, and challenge insurance companies who will not pay for therapies that they believe are not evidence-based. This empowerment can result in greater understanding and acceptance of fibromyalgia, increased optimism about the condition, and a more positive mood and outlook.[360, 361] Someone with fibromyalgia may feel a sense of community and sustenance by interacting with others who experience the symptoms and encounter identical difficulties. Moreover, sharing solutions can be a focus of group interactions, as creative ideas are bounced around and analyzed and further improved with multiple inputs. An appropriate group may be recommended through your family physician or a group may be found on the world-wide web (Internet) through an online search. Also, churches and recreation departments may be able to provide transportation to or facilities for such events.

❖ Cognitive Therapy

Like awareness groups and self-help organizations, talking to professionals in the form of formalized therapy has been explored for improving fibromyalgia. Specifically, cognitive therapy, which is a type of psychotherapy that focuses on a client's perception and interpretation (cognition) of life events. The idea behind cognitive therapy is that errors in the thought process contributed to psychological problems. For example, in the context of cognitive therapy, the tendency to magnify the negative aspects of life could keep someone depressed; thus, correcting these errors in thinking (and thereby eliminating the negative thought pattern) could influence emotions and reverse the depression.

Cognitive therapy applied to fibromyalgia suggests that giving people positive thoughts about their illness could decrease their physical symptoms and improve their health. This is especially important considering that people with fibromyalgia have amplified physical responses to stimuli which may manifest as an outsized stress response, and cognitive therapy could re-align these responses.

In some studies, scientists found that cognitive therapy was not helpful for people with fibromyalgia and was expensive.[362, 363] Other studies have yielded results that suggest cognitive therapy was useful in teaching patients coping skills and methods for altering their response to stress which could be used in future pain episodes.[364, 365]

A common thread in the argument for receiving effective help for fibromyalgia is that people who do not have this disease simply cannot understand it. This very concept may be the difference between positive and negative outcomes in therapeutic processes. Perhaps some studies were not positive because the therapist did not understand what someone who suffers from fibromyalgia endures, so he was less empathetic. Such differences in understanding and experience might be significant enough to skew the results of such therapy. For example, perhaps the catastrophizing (the act of emphasizing an almost irrational negativity) and depressive self-statements made by the study participants were regarded as extreme or unrealistic by study directors or therapists who could not visualize the suffering. After all, how could someone so apparently able-bodied be so down in the dumps! Because the therapists had likely not dealt with days and months of unrelenting pain and fatigue, they simply could not identify with the problems described by people with fibromyalgia.

Outrageous Claims

Although many massage therapists, acupuncturists, and yoga instructors are well-trained in their discipline, the best practitioners within these fields will be cautious not to overstep their training. Unscrupulous practitioners who deliberately exceed the limits of their knowledge—often for financial gain—can cause confusion at best, and great harm at worst, when they attempt to diagnose, prescribe, or treat people with fibromyalgia or when they make false claims. For example, I have received unsolicited and false advice from several people who practice these disciplines. Happily, my scientific background helps me ignore any bad information that I receive. However, for people who may not have such training, such potentially harmful advice may actually sound terrific or sensible.

I cannot recall each crazy claim made by people who have offered advice to me, but I can list the most ridiculous things I have heard in the past and refute them here. Hopefully, these ideas will give you a healthy skepticism of people who do not have a scientific background, but instead may have training in aesthetics, massage therapy, or acupuncture. Of note, a bachelor's degree is not considered by experts to be a sufficient scientific background, but it is a suitable foundation for future training and expertise.

Claim: Fibromyalgia is due to toxins.

Response: We do not produce toxins, which are biologically made poisons. We may be *exposed* to toxins (snake venom, plant-based poisons) or to toxicants, which are poisons that are not biological in origin, and specific antidotes exist for many poisonings. Nevertheless, exposure to a particular toxin or toxicant has not been shown to cause fibromyalgia.

For those concerned about our daily exposures to strange substances in foods, drugs, and the environment, you should know that most healthy individuals can eliminate the small amounts of unwanted compounds that we encounter. For example, our liver, kidneys, and other organs routinely and safely detoxify and/or metabolize drugs we ingest. Then, we excrete this degraded material via the urine and feces. So, unless we work in industrial areas and have occupational exposures to dangerous compounds, we should not worry too much about toxicants and how to remove them from our bodies.

Claim: Soy products have caused your fibromyalgia.

Response: The peer-reviewed literature does not support this claim, and soy may be beneficial for some people who cannot tolerate or must avoid meat sources of protein. Unless you have a soy allergy or you are being treated for certain cancers that can be affected by estrogen, you do not have to avoid soy.

Claim: Metal toxicity caused your fibromyalgia.

Response: Metal toxicity, such as lead or mercury poisoning, is a serious concern, and subsequent actual metal toxicities must be treated according to specific guidelines. Still, exposures to metals in sufficient quantities to pose a problem is quite rare outside of occupational exposures. Either way, metals have not been shown to cause fibromyalgia.

Claim: Your fatigue is due to accumulation of waste/food/material in your colon.

Response: True, bloating and constipation can make you fell less than peppy, but you never *need* colonics, colon cleansing, or enemas unless medically prescribed for colonoscopy preparation or similar treatments. Eat fiber and drink water to regulate your body instead of taking a harsh, back-door approach. If you have a serious stomach or intestinal disorder like diverticulitis, persistent reflux, or blockage, seek medical attention.

Claim: Artificial sweeteners and non-organic foods cause your fibromyalgia.

Response: This idea is not supported by the scientific literature. Artificial sweeteners are safe and they are excellent substitutes for table sugar when you want to reduce calories. No artificial sweetener approved by the US FDA has been shown to be carcinogenic in humans or harmful in recommended amounts.

Also, at this time, organic foods and products are not more nutritious for you than conventionally grown foods. The quality of the soil greatly determines nutritional content of food. Moreover, washing all produce in running water before eating the food essentially removes residues of pesticides and chemicals. Remember that natural is not necessarily safer: after all, cyanide and arsenic are natural, too.

Claim: If you take these vitamins or supplements that I sell, you will get rid of your fibromyalgia.

Response: Science does not support the idea that vitamin deficiencies cause fibromyalgia. Thus, adding vitamins supplements to your diet is not considered beneficial for specifically reducing fibromyalgia symptoms. Striving for nutritionally complete meals is ideal, and some supplements can round out a diet that is less than perfect. Be wary of spas and health care professional who formulate and sell their own supplements to make a profit. Most supplements or vitamins just create expensive urine. If your diet is varied and healthful, you do not need additional pills.

In conclusion, do not believe everything you hear, and be skeptical of anyone who claims to be able to cure fibromyalgia. At this time, there is no proven cure for fibromyalgia, but symptoms can be improved with healthy lifestyles and exercise, perhaps complemented with prescribed drug therapies for some individuals.

Chapter Summary

- ❖ Drugs may not be suitable for people with fibromyalgia for various reasons.
- ❖ Non-drug treatment options are attractive to people with fibromyalgia because they may cost less and have fewer risks.
- ❖ Active participation activities are excellent for reducing pain and fatigue and controlling weight.
- ❖ Passive participation activities can be relaxing and may reduce pain and fatigue and improve sleep.
- ❖ Combining both active and passive activities can surpass the benefit of choosing only one type of method for controlling fibromyalgia.

❖ Beware of people who tell you outlandish things to "cure" your fibromyalgia or who want to sell you something to improve your symptoms, and always react to any new information with healthy skepticism.

CHAPTER 6—FOR PEOPLE WHO SUPPORT OTHERS WITH FIBROMYALGIA

Supporting Someone with Fibromyalgia?

If someone you know has fibromyalgia, the first fact your friend or loved one would want you to know is that *fibromyalgia is a very real condition*. Fibromyalgia is as authentic as any disease that overwhelms an individual and impairs his functional ability, potentially leading to depression, despair, or further disability. Because the pain of fibromyalgia cannot be cured, the person afflicted with this condition can only manage the symptoms or modify their life to accommodate the problem. You should also know that the person you support with fibromyalgia is grateful for your assistance, kindness, and willingness to travel this path with him or her.

❖ Encountering Beliefs about Fibromyalgia

For a long time, physicians who encountered people with fibromyalgia doubted the legitimacy of fibromyalgia as a real disease and an explanation for aches, fatigue, and mental fogginess. In fact, the scientific and medical literature includes earlier articles which describe this initial disbelief by physicians and other medical professionals.[366-374] Although more than 20 years have passed since the first descriptions of fibromyalgia, and much clinical work has been done to characterize this illness, the actual acceptance of fibromyalgia as a *unique and real clinical disorder* is constantly being challenged. First, the greatest doubt about fibromyalgia being real arises from the entirely subjective nature of pain. Pain is felt differently by individuals, so perception of pain varies widely. Thus, the very idea of painful tender points is suspect.

Interestingly, older people with fibromyalgia report different issues with fibromyalgia than younger people with the condition. Scientists suggest that more mature sufferers have adapted to their problem and have used adult problem-solving techniques to manage their condition.[375, 376] In contrast, younger people are more prone to viewing chronic pain and fatigue as more disruptive to their lives, as they may never have experienced age-related declines in health. Therefore, younger, healthy people may have more negative viewpoints about their condition, ideas that are fueled by their expectations of a long, pain-free, and virtually unencumbered life. Older adults can bring diverse experiences into their interpretations that translate into wisdoms, which can ultimately lower their frustrations regarding pain, illness, and suffering. Thus, fibromyalgia may not be viewed as particularly devastating by older people who have such perspectives.[376]

Also, there is apparently no reliable biomarker of fibromyalgia that is consistent in all people who report having the illness, which further complicates ideas about fibromyalgia. Most commonly, markers or indicators of disease and health can be measured in body fluids like blood or urine. For a fibromyalgia biomarker to be useful and conclusive, the biomarker would be present in the blood or urine of all fibromyalgia sufferers, and ideally the biomarker would be greater or more abundant in people who have more severe fibromyalgia. Likewise, anyone who did not have fibromyalgia could not show signs of the biomarker. More about this is covered in Chapter 2, §Reliable Laboratory Tests.

Laboratory tests aside, even now—after much research into fibromyalgia and the approval of three drugs to treat it—some medical professionals do not accept the idea of fibromyalgia as a real disease. Perhaps this is due to ignorance on behalf of the clinician, suspicion of the patient, or simply an honest misunderstanding of the information in the scientific literature.[368, 370, 377] Interestingly, the scientific literature suggests that the strongest arguments against the claim of fibromyalgia being real come from health insurance companies and employers who purchase or subsidize the health insurance, who have financial interests in payment for medical services, drugs, and disability claims from employers.[370, 372, 377, 378] Thus, this bias and lack of acceptance of fibromyalgia as a real disease is often financially motivated.

❖ Relating to People with Fibromyalgia

Thus, people with fibromyalgia are accustomed to others minimizing or discounting their pain or fatigue. In fact, such dismissal of their symptoms can become a continual theme in the life of a fibromyalgia sufferer. Because no one can *see* the disability, it is easy for others to say that it is not real or that it is not so terrible. Some people with fibromyalgia have been asked to "unlearn their disability conviction", suggesting that they can decide to be well as easily as they "decided" to be ill.[379] Fibromyalgia is often a double curse for this reason: they are in pain and tired, and they may have shame because they are treated like frauds.[366]

Guilt is also associated with fibromyalgia.[366, 380] Not only do people with fibromyalgia feel exhausted and ill, but also they often feel guilty for needing so much extra time, help, comfort, space, etc. From this guilt can arise feelings of despair and sadness or depression. [381]In fact, depression is reported with fibromyalgia in 50–70% of cases.[55] [33] Likely this phenomenon is under-documented because many people do not realize that they have fibromyalgia and do not seek treatment or they believe that they feel bad because they are depressed, not realizing that they may have two problems.[382]

Depression often mimics the symptoms of fibromyalgia, and fibromyalgia can cause people to feel depressed about their situation.[55, 383] People with fibromyalgia and depression may be difficult to interact and live with. Negativity, catastrophizing (taking extremely negative viewpoints), helplessness and general pessimism may accompany fibromyalgia and these feelings could be attributed to the sufferer's opinion about the lack of control he has over the problem.[384-386] Interestingly, medicine and science have concentrated on the one aspect of controlling fibromyalgia symptoms—such as exercise and drugs—and have focused less on a holistic mind-body approach to this disorder. Thus, research is generally lacking on ideas to address mood in fibromyalgia.[384]

One way to meet the needs of someone with fibromyalgia who exhibits depressive tendencies is to listen with detachment (do not take what you are hearing as a personal assault) but with sympathy. Offering emotional support is useful and this includes showing understanding, patience, and encouragement. Listening carefully and actively is a good idea. When inviting a loved one with fibromyalgia for walks, outings, and other activities, it is fine to be gently insistent in the face of initial refusals, but do not push the individual. As important as diversion and company may be, the person with fibromyalgia is attuned to the fact that he has turned down multiple offers for companionship and worsen any feelings of failure.

Depression associated with fibromyalgia can take turn dark corners, potentially leading to drug addiction and alcoholism. Sometimes, people find that a drink or two in the evening decreases their tension and pain, but over time, tolerance to alcohol can develop. Thus, a person must drink more to feel the same relaxation. Because alcohol damages the liver over time, this can lead to life-threatening problems if it continues for a significant length of time.

Also, if the person you support with fibromyalgia takes medication, drinking and taking drugs can be dangerous. If you suspect that your friend or family member with fibromyalgia is developing a substance-abuse problem, you may want to suggest that he get professional help. Problems such as these often require the assistance of trained professionals, and many people who support someone with fibromyalgia may not have the capacity or resources to help someone with a drug or drinking problem.

❖ **Helpful Ideas to Support People with Fibromyalgia**

Gift certificates for massage therapy or acupuncture (please ask first) may be welcome. Also, a few hours of housework offered to someone with fibromyalgia who cannot manage household chores and tasks alone can be very kind. For someone with children, a willingness to babysit for an afternoon can be a dear asset to one with fibromyalgia who needs a quiet break from the kids.

As you may have guessed, people with fibromyalgia can have variable response to touch. Simply hugging a person with fibromyalgia can bring her to tears. Children who bump and jostle a person with fibromyalgia can further isolate that person because he already feels terrible, and having to withdraw from family activities to avoid painful interactions can be even more distressing. Because being social can be such a burden, people with fibromyalgia may refuse invitations for trips, vacations, outings, and similar activities to avoid explanations. Often, these refusals can, over time, destroy social networks and wreak unpredictable personal havoc on the mind and body. Thus, to help someone with fibromyalgia who might experience these symptoms, you may want to refrain from hugging them and offer a handshake instead. Also, asking children to be more gentle or less boisterous can be helpful to the person with chronic pain.

Because fibromyalgia can make normal errands unappealing, perhaps you can offer to return books that are due to the library, or to take the dog for a walk, water house plants, or rake leaves. Alternately, you can occasionally suggest picking up dry cleaning or something for dinner for someone with fibromyalgia. Chances are excellent that something that you do without thinking about it is a challenge for someone with fibromyalgia. Thus, many times help is often welcome and greatly appreciated.

If you live with someone with fibromyalgia, opening jars and cans for that person is a wonderful treat. Often, grip strength is weak in people with fibromyalgia, and twisting stubborn jar lids is painful. Chopping vegetables, tearing salad greens, and helping in the kitchen are wonderful ways to enjoy company and conversation while being helpful.

While it is true that a few people will use fibromyalgia as an excuse not to participate in anything physical, most people do not use their fibromyalgia as a wall to keep away people and joyful interactions. Rather, fibromyalgia sufferers are grateful for patience and kindness, coupled with understanding. If someone with fibromyalgia refuses an invitation to an event, ask again at a different time.

If possible, the activities you suggest for the person with fibromyalgia should be directed at enabling them to have power over their symptoms. Exercise can be part of that plan. If you can take walks or short bicycle rides with the person, this would be ideal. Often the company provided is worth the initial energy it might take to begin the walk. Ideally, the person with fibromyalgia will be enjoying the activity to the degree that he does feel better and this will make subsequent attempts to exercise easy.

❖ Ideas to Avoid for People with Fibromyalgia

People with fibromyalgia can have trouble just getting through the day. Unlike the flu, fibromyalgia does not go away after a week, and there is no escape from the annoying symptoms that are part of the disorder. What can make the whole problem worse is to hear that the pain of fibromyalgia is also a pain and burden to someone else. Minimizing the tiredness ("How can you be tired? You just woke up!") or expressing frustration over something that a person with fibromyalgia cannot control ("But you always say your back hurts!") can destroy communication.

Patience is required to live a life with fibromyalgia, but more than patience is needed to be a positive and helpful supporter of someone with fibromyalgia. Accusing someone with fibromyalgia of faking the illness or laziness or expecting him/her to get over it is not helpful. If possible, do not disparage any feelings expressed by the person with fibromyalgia, but subtly point out realities and try to offer hope. Never ignore remarks about suicide, but seek professional help if this occurs.

❖ Professional Help

Naturally, there will be a limit to what you can do for someone, especially if that person will not help himself. This is regrettable but common. When you feel that you have no more to offer or that the person with fibromyalgia is experiencing a downward spiral in attitude or health, professional intervention may be in order. If you have clergy who are trusted and available, this might be a route for you. If you can suggest or make physician appointments for the person you support, this also might be a good thing to do. Overall, emphasize that you are reaching out to alternate sources because you care not because you have given up. We are not all trained to handle complex issues such as supporting others with illnesses, and it is perfectly fine to admit your limitation and seek answers elsewhere. Often the best sign of a smart supporter is not that he knows all the answers but that he can go find the answer form someone else.

Non-drug treatments are discussed in great detail in the previous Chapter, and these might be suitable recommendations for the person you support. Keep in mind the preferences of your friend or loved one when suggesting yoga, massage, or a support group. A few people have an aversion to being touched by strangers, so a massage treatment may be out of the question. Also, the friend with a poor self-image may not be ready for yoga, and may find the prospect of a gym membership for exercise more stressful than being tired and in pain.

A support group is not recommended for those who experience stress when listening to stories about fibromyalgia symptoms. Certainly, some individuals may not relate to this type of sharing, may find the experience uncomfortable, may perceive the group members as whiny or complaining, or may not want to focus on their condition so much. Some people specifically enjoy the company of others who do not have fibromyalgia because they can emphasize other aspects of life instead of their condition. There are a few people who also resist the idea of having their fibromyalgia diagnosed, thereby giving a name to their symptoms. These people imagine that having a true diagnosis somehow makes them more "ill" and causes them to perceive their health in a more negative light. Thus, if you support

❖ Fibromyalgia as a Disability

Fibromyalgia can result in disability which can increase the sense of helplessness and defeat, especially if a job loss results in an unstable financial situation.[387-390] In surveys of people with fibromyalgia, almost half report losing their job because of their illness.[391] Whether fibromyalgia rises to the level of disability for someone is an individual determination. Some people can work a regular job and muddle through life's chores with fibromyalgia. Others simply cannot, and their condition imposes a disability. In fact, up to 25% of people seen in rheumatology clinics for fibromyalgia and related disorders have received some type of disability compensation.[392]

The Americans with Disabilities Act (ADA) of 1990 protects people with disabilities in the workforce and applies to any business that has more than 15 employees. Under the ADA, a person with a disability is defined as "a person who has a physical or mental impairment that substantially limits one or more major life activities, has a record of such an impairment, or is regarded as having such an impairment."[393]

The key to this definition is that persons so defined must have real impairments that include limitations to performing manual tasks, caring for oneself, and working. The ADA also distinguishes between short-term injuries which are not covered and long-term, present conditions. Thus, cancer in remission would not be covered. The crux of this definition and the protection it provides is demonstrating that fibromyalgia is a real condition of long-term duration. Being classified as disabled is important to people with fibromyalgia, if the severity of their symptoms warrant such classification. Social Security Disability Insurance is provided to workers who become disabled to the degree that they are unable to maintain gainful employment. The Insurance, or Disability payments are provided to assure that the disability does not cause the disabled individual to become impoverished.

Fibromyalgia falls under the category of subjective claims, which means that your employer must rely on the employee's reporting of the disability. This complicates matters for employers because recently, disability claims for subjective issues such as fatigue an pain have increased as the stress of the workforce and economic troubles bear down on everyone.[394] An employer cannot reasonably determine which of these disability claims are legitimate or whether they arise from a disease or common stressors.[395] This creates a higher burden of proof for the person with fibromyalgia who must not only demonstrate having the condition to a disabling degree but who must also prove that fibromyalgia is real.[366] The complexity of characterizing fibromyalgia as a disability that should exempt the sufferer from employment rests with the concept that physical activity is beneficial for people with fibromyalgia. Movement decreased pain and fatigue and promotes feelings of well being. Certainly, the loss of a job would compound the depression that may accompany fibromyalgia. Thus, it would seem that work or gainful employment would be a form of treatment.

Chapter Summary

❖ Fibromyalgia is a real, persistent condition.

❖ Kindness and patience are good attributes of people who provide support to those with fibromyalgia.

❖ There is no reliable biomarker for the presence or severity of fibromyalgia.

❖ Health care providers, employers, and insurers may not accept the idea that fibromyalgia is a real illness.

❖ Fibromyalgia feels differently to different people.

❖ People with fibromyalgia may feel guilt and may experience depression.

❖ Listening and offering emotional support is useful.

❖ People with fibromyalgia may respond negatively to touch.

❖ Fibromyalgia can lead people to decline social invitations.

❖ Help with chores or errands may be a good idea.

❖ Offering companionship during light exercise may be helpful.

❖ Minimizing symptoms is not helpful.

❖ Professional help can be recommended for unworkable situations.

❖ Fibromyalgia can lead to disability if the impairment rises to the level defined by the Americans with Disabilities Act.

Chapter 7—
Fibromyalgia in
Children

Can Fibromyalgia be Diagnosed in Youth?

The current medical and scientific literature chiefly focuses on adults when describing fibromyalgia symptoms and treatments. However, the first description of juvenile fibromyalgia appeared in 1985, and new information is continually emerging about this condition, indicating that children indeed experience fibromyalgia symptoms, and that they can be diagnosed with fibromyalgia.[396, 397] For children with fibromyalgia, the symptoms are similar to those for adults: muscle pain, headaches, unrefreshing sleep, and lack of focus.[396, 398] Also, some physicians agree that 5 tender points in children are sufficient for a fibromyalgia diagnosis—instead of the customary 11 out of 18 tender points—if the other supporting symptoms are present.[399]

Such confirmation can be comforting to parents of children who have these symptoms because they finally have a name for what is going on. Sadly, often such complaints from children are dismissed as "growing pains", or the parents become fearful that their child's symptoms are evidence of a more serious or life-threatening disease.[264] Thus, a diagnosis of juvenile fibromyalgia—which is fibromyalgia occurring in people younger than 17 years-of-age—is gaining greater acceptance in the medical community.[396] This means that more research is being directed toward younger sufferers. In fact, the FIQ (Chapter 3) has been modified for children, and new treatment strategies for this population are under investigation.[400]

❖ Gender Differences

Interestingly, boys and girls with juvenile fibromyalgia have similar symptoms, and boys appear to be equally affected as girls. Also, as boys mature, fibromyalgia symptoms seem to disappear in many, almost spontaneously. Scientist suggest that such differences between boys and girls could be explained by hormones which can pay a role in the duration and severity of fibromyalgia.[92] Some researchers have suggested that young girls share a disproportionate prevalence of fibromyalgia may complain more of fibromyalgia symptoms because of behavioral conditioning by one parent who has fibromyalgia, usually the mother because of the adult prevalence of fibromyalgia being greater in women. Thus, the parent models a particular behavior, and the daughter adopts this behavior, so daughters may be simply mimicking their mothers with fibromyalgia.

Studies to investigate whether young girls have fibromyalgia or are simply "sympathizing" with their mothers revealed that the symptoms were indeed real. No differences in psychological well-being were detected in families with histories of adult and juvenile fibromyalgia. Also, daughters of mothers with fibromyalgia reported similar symptoms even if they lived away from the parent with fibromyalgia.[92]

Having diagnostic criteria for children with fibromyalgia as well as an awareness that this disorder exists in juveniles is critical because children who present to physicians with fatigue, muscular pain, and headaches often undergo invasive and unnecessary testing to rule out other diseases.[396] Perhaps with a greater understanding of the prevalence of fibromyalgia in young persons, diagnoses can be made more quickly for this population and with fewer false starts that are inconvenient for both parents and children, and ultimately and unnecessarily drive up the cost of health care.

Accepting that fibromyalgia can occur in children also challenges the idea that fibromyalgia need arise from a physical or psychological stress because many of children diagnosed with fibromyalgia are likely (hopefully) too young to have experienced such traumas. Supporting this idea is the fact that little or no evidence was found for such stresses in young people with fibromyalgia. Rather, these children were generally more sensitive—and perhaps always had been—to stimuli than their peers who did not have fibromyalgia.[145] Thus, one might conclude that no specific triggering event is needed for the onset of fibromyalgia, either in children or adults. Perhaps the predisposition to have ultra-receptive senses is present at birth and exacerbated by traumas and related events. An interesting study might be to explore the temperament of children early in life and learn whether infants ultra-sensitive to light, sound, and touch eventually matured into children (and then adults) with fibromyalgia. To date, such studies have not been conducted.

❖ Obesity and Fibromyalgia

Because US children are increasingly becoming a significant share of the US obesity epidemic, it is important to understand the connection, if any, between obesity and fibromyalgia. Exercise intolerance and fatigue can discourage children from playing and moving, which may cause weight gain in normal weight children or worsen existing weight problems in juveniles who are already obese.[401] Childhood obesity is defined as having a body weight in excess of 20% above ideal weight for age and gender and skin-fold thickness.[402, 403] Because most parents may not know the ideal body weight for their child's age, this information can also be found on pediatric percentile charts. These instruments can be found by using an Internet search engine and entering "pediatric or adolescent percentile height and weight charts". Some libraries may also have reference books that include these types of charts, and a librarian can help you find this information. Using these charts, an obese child will have a weight above the 85th percentile for that child's age and gender.[402, 403]

Scientists have reported that children who are overweight do have more musculoskeletal complaints.[404] Also, in children who experienced significant weight loss after being obese, the number of musculoskeletal problems decreased.[401, 405] This result was also reported in studies including adults: weight reduction in overweight people with fibromyalgia was correlated to symptom improvement.[406] This might suggest that any muscular pain experienced overweight children is simply because they are heavy. Thus, problems of overweight children should be discounted or ignored because such issues can be resolved with a diet and exercise plan that promotes weight loss. A more practical approach may be for the physician or caregiver to accept that an overweight or obese child can absolutely have fibromyalgia, and that the extra weight may aggravate the symptoms. Therefore, weight loss alone may not eliminate every symptoms.

Any parent embarking on a plan to reduce a child's weight to alleviate symptoms of fibromyalgia must be cautious and ensure that the plan has three approaches: the plan should be healthy; the plan should be calorically appropriate; sufficient exercise should be included; and behavior management supported by the whole family should be a component. A treatment plan for an obese child that is managed by a heavy parent can be confusing to the child and difficult to enforce.

Thus, an overweight or obese parent must be honestly introspective and consider whether both the child and parent should attempt the weight loss and exercise plan together.

Aside from obesity, dietary considerations may be important for children with fibromyalgia. Studies in children with rheumatoid arthritis indicated that vegetarian diets improved symptoms, but this was attributed to avoiding foods that previously increased inflammation in the study subjects.[407] Because fibromyalgia is not an inflammatory disease, modified diets may not be helpful for many children in this regard. Nevertheless, a healthy diet that is moderate to low in saturated fat, high in fruits and vegetables, and low in sugar may improve mood in addition to helping a child maintain a healthy, stable body weight. These positive effects may contribute to an increased ability to cope with fibromyalgia.

❖ Adequate Rest in Juvenile Fibromyalgia

Sleep is important to the health of normal children, and especially those children with fibromyalgia, which can interfere with sleep. Research into children with fibromyalgia also suggests that excessive limb movement during sleep contributes to diminished restorative rest.[408] These children with restless limbs awakened more often in the night and took much longer to fall asleep. A child who cannot sleep and recharge after a full day of school and play is significantly disadvantaged when compared to young people who are able to receive sufficient rest each night. In fact, juvenile fibromyalgia is associated with poor concentration at school.[264] Such lack of focus might be attributed to being poorly rested, which puts a child at risk for falling asleep during school and encountering disciplinary measures for this misinterpreted "laziness". Of course, like adults, fibromyalgia symptoms and the child's response to these can spill over and potentially negatively influence other areas of life.

Studies including people with chronic pain conditions such as fibromyalgia often experience anxiety, hopelessness, and suicidal thoughts. For teens and pre-teens, this is a complicated picture because simply being a teenager can be a challenge. Teen years are legendary times for feeling unattractive, unaccepted, and detached from peer groups. This temporary angst coupled with fibromyalgia may be a tipping point for certain susceptible personalities. Children with fibromyalgia report increased anxiety, stress, and depression.[145] Thus, extra care should be taken with some juveniles when supporting them and teaching them coping skills for their fibromyalgia.

So, not only can fibromyalgia be difficult for the individual child to face, friendships can be affected in children with fibromyalgia. Interesting research into social relationships among juveniles with fibromyalgia suggest that children with these symptoms have difficulty making and maintaining friendships, and were more frequently described as withdrawn, both by their peers and by their own reports.[145, 409]

Furthermore, children with fibromyalgia are reported to miss more school that their healthy counterparts.[410] Such scholastic obstacles can increase the negativity associated with fatigue and pain, and this can present an insurmountable barrier to juveniles who lack positive parental input and emotional support. Possibly, an appropriate and pro-active approach to helping a child with fibromyalgia may be to contact the school or teacher to explain the condition and symptoms. Frequently, schools will request health information for each enrolled child to monitor medications and allergies. This health information form might be a perfect place to indicate that your child has fibromyalgia. Here you can list the specific symptoms your child experiences and mention the triggers or stressors that seem to make the situation worse.

If a pediatrician or family practitioner diagnosed your child with fibromyalgia, a note from either one of these specialists can be helpful for informing the school about your child's specific needs. Surely, a teacher would be gratified to know the source of the problem and be willing to grant leniency with your child during trying times. Teachers, who are often inherently curious and open-minded, can be significant allies in providing support for your child at school. Also, the principal or headmaster might be able to offer guidance.

❖ Juvenile Fibromyalgia and Families

Fibromyalgia changes how children interact with parents, and this can be enhanced or diminished by the responses parents offer to these children in such interactions.[145] When researchers evaluated the parent-child relationship in children with fibromyalgia, some unique findings emerged. First, children who had positive parental support when they performed mildly fatiguing exercises fared better than children whose parents discouraged them from coping with the exertion.[410] In contrast, when parents encouraged coping skills, the children performed better and for longer periods of time during mildly painful activities. Also, in a study to evaluate parents of children with fibromyalgia who also had a history of chronic pain conditions, a correlation was found between parents who coped well with their chronic pain and their children's coping ability: the better the parent managed pain, the healthier their child's attitude was toward this stressful condition.[411] Thus, coping and pain management can be taught.

Similar to research findings with adults, exercise is thought to benefit children with fibromyalgia.[90, 264] Physical education classes during school can address some of the exercise, especially if the movement is continual and adequately aerobic. Sports with frequent breaks and idle moments such as basketball, volleyball, and baseball might not be sufficiently vigorous for controlling fibromyalgia symptoms. However, running, walking, and more interactive sports like gymnastics and soccer may provide more relief. Thus, exercise is a highly acceptable form of therapy for juvenile fibromyalgia. Having a parent suggest, encourage, or even participate in the exercise might be a way to improve parent-child interactions and have both get some exercise.

Also, cognitive and occupational therapy have been suggested for people with juvenile fibromyalgia.[412] Occupational therapists are professionals trained to assist people of all ages in improving their ability to perform tasks of daily living and working such as dressing, cooking, feeding oneself. Drug treatment for juvenile fibromyalgia is also being investigated. Cyclobenzaprine (See Chapter 4) is reported to be helpful for juvenile fibromyalgia.[264] Antidepressants have also been used in small numbers of patients with positive results.[413] Researchers also suggest that medications proven to be helpful in adults with fibromyalgia hold promise for juvenile sufferers of fibromyalgia, but studies are too early in development to draw conclusions at this time.

An intriguing suggestion emerging from juvenile fibromyalgia studies is that some children may outgrow the symptoms of fibromyalgia. In fact, some children with fibromyalgia have been reported to have so few symptoms of fibromyalgia that they no longer can be classified as having the disorder.

Chapter Summary

- ❖ Juvenile fibromyalgia symptoms are similar to adult symptoms.
- ❖ A specific trauma might not be necessary for fibromyalgia in children, and perhaps in adults.
- ❖ Fibromyalgia in children may be attributed to an over-sensing predisposition of the nervous system.
- ❖ Juvenile fibromyalgia can negatively affect activities at school, relationships with peers, and interactions with parents.
- ❖ Exercise is an accepted therapy for fibromyalgia in children.
- ❖ Some drugs used with success in adults may hold promise in children.

❖ Parental support with coping skills has been shown to be positive for children with fibromyalgia.

❖ Scientists speculate that some children, boys in particular, with fibromyalgia may outgrow their symptoms.

Chapter 8—My Experience with Fibromyalgia

When I tell people that I have fibromyalgia, most do not believe me immediately. After all, I seem to be reasonably fit and healthy, without any apparent physical problems. Because fibromyalgia is a disease of altered perception to pain, which is a highly personal and virtually invisible experience, no one knows how I feel unless I vocalize my discomfort. In fact, only my immediate family really knows what I have to manage every day. So, on the very rare occasion that the topic of fibromyalgia comes up in conversation—or under the more unique circumstance that I actually reveal that I have fibromyalgia—people who are familiar with fibromyalgia as a chronic condition inevitably tell me that my situation "is not so bad" or they ask me what I do to seem so "normal".

To address this important question comprehensively, this Chapter is devoted to describing my experience with fibromyalgia, as well as offering a glimpse into my personal routine to manage my fibromyalgia. Please remember that I have been "working at" fibromyalgia management for more than half of my life, and I have tried—and frustratingly discarded—more ideas than I have adopted. Therefore, I hope my trials and errors might be useful as you look for solutions for yourself.

Of course, if you are newly diagnosed with fibromyalgia, you may be overwhelmed with the concept of trying anything new, believing that you will never be ready to make drastic changes—you simply do not have the energy! If that is the case, this Chapter may temporarily discourage you. On the other hand, perhaps my story will make you laugh and relax somewhat about your condition, and maybe you will see additional possibilities for yourself. Perhaps you will be energized to attempt something you read here, or you will be motivated to change a nagging habit that you know is not helpful for you. Either way, I hope that this Chapter will inspire you to think differently, and perhaps positively, about fibromyalgia.

Twenty Years and Still Hanging in There

I have had fibromyalgia for as along as I can recall, perhaps as far back as 13 years-of-age. As a teen, I was tired all of the time, and simple exertion felt like a monumental effort. I literally dragged and sagged through my classes in school, through band practice, through babysitting...you name it, I moped through it like a wet rag. When I could get away with it, I would sleep for days. I was literally unable to wake up. When I did force myself to get out of the bed, I was foggy for the entire day and utterly useless. In the evening, I was relieved to go back to sleep, giving up again on another day. My family's interpretation of my habits was that I was going through a lazy phase, or that I was just being a teenager.

Later, through college and graduate school, my sleep habits worsened: I was a light sleeper, awake at any noise, and I never felt rested, ever. In college, I lived in a noisy dormitory, and much of my sleeplessness was attributed to the lousy environment. During the day, my life was not much better, as I sat for hours per week in classes and in the laboratory.

Eventually, I realized that I was not moving much during the day, and I guessed that this might have something to do with my perpetual exhaustion. To test this idea, I experimented with walking at night to get away from the noise in the dorm, and to have some time to myself. I found that not only was the walking very tolerable, but it was enjoyable, giving me time to listen to music on my headphones while I toured the neighborhoods around the campus. I also realized over time that this exercise was making me more tired at night, and I actually fell asleep now and then during the week, in spite of the noisy dorm. Another benefit of so much walking was that my weight finally became stable, a frustration I had poorly managed since I was thirteen.

In my twenties, I found a name for my problem: fibromyalgia. With this new knowledge, and my constant quest for information about the topic, I was able to recognize other symptoms that I had, which were reported to be prevalent for people with fibromyalgia. For example, in addition to constant, nagging pain and sleepiness, I had continual irritable bowel syndrome (IBS) that I have learned to manage with diet and exercise. Also, I had multiple numb areas on my back and shoulders that appeared in my early twenties, with no apparent explanation. My visit to a neurologist about these numb areas was not particularly illuminating; the physician remarked that many women my age complained of mysterious numb patches. He offered no rationale for my experience, and he suggested I ignore it. As I reached my thirties, I noticed that I was becoming increasingly intolerant to cold, and that when I did spend any time in cold weather, my hands and feet became numb and they seemed to "burn" when I came inside to warm up. I felt like I was aging twice as fast as anyone else.

Now, I now that my numb areas on my back are paresthesias, and I understand that my reaction to cold weather was Reynaud's Syndrome, which is predictable for me when the temperature drops to only 60 °F. I now accept that my fingers and toes will blanch and become completely numb for about 30 minutes after the cold exposure. I have learned to tolerate this because it is only a problem in winter, which is mild where I presently live, or when my family goes skiing in the mountains out west.

The other symptoms that I have which I now associate with fibromyalgia are not so difficult for me anymore: IBS, frequent trips to the restroom, having to shift in my chair dozens of times a day because my legs and back hurt constantly, etc. In fact, at this time, I really only have one problem that wipes me out: unrefreshing sleep. For example, I may make it through the week with 2 hours of sleep each night. I can pull this off for a few weeks, and no one would guess that this is all of the rest I get. By the end of the week, I am usually so exhausted that I do fall asleep for up to 4 hours. Still, this is not optimal, and it represents a significant challenge for me.

Because sleep is such a luxury that I so desperately seek, I once attempted to enroll in an insomnia study that was being conducted by a clinical laboratory in my town. I was excited at the prospect of being evaluated and perhaps being treated for a condition I had fought for so long. I happily filled out the paperwork for the study and documented, as requested, the time I went to bed, the time I awoke, the time it took me to fall asleep, along with every instance of being awake during the night. Imagine my surprise when I got a call from the study coordinator who regretted to inform me that I didn't sleep enough to qualify for the insomnia study! I had to laugh...because crying took too much energy.

Even with fibromyalgia and all of the symptoms that go with it, I still work full-time, parent full-time, and run my house and personal life the rest of the time. I do not have a personal assistant, personal trainer, chef, or nanny, and any help I could have from my relatives is a full day away by car. Thus, I am on my own when it comes to everyday tasks.

Still, over time, I have decided that I can largely direct my own life script, incorporating and managing good habits to improve my life instead of flaking out, being lazy, and letting my fibromyalgia dictate that I adopt bad habits that will increase my pain, fatigue, and other symptoms and ultimately diminish my joyful moments. Hopefully, this final Chapter will give you a glimpse into what I do to *make it through* the day as well as *enjoy* the day, and maybe you will laugh a little, too.

My Life with Fibromyalgia

First, my family has graciously accepted that my fibromyalgia makes me a little nutty. This minor frailty (and it is only that...it is not terminal) of mine has caused a few mishaps that we still laugh about. Here are some of my stories about what my fibromyalgia has done to me, and by extension, to my family:

❖ Old Lady Disease

My daughter and my husband, who are compassionate and kind souls, know that I deal with fatigue and pain every day, but this does not make them reconsider what they will have me do on vacation. For instance, on our annual pilgrimage to the ski slopes of Utah or Colorado, we did as we traditionally do as a family—ski for several hours every day when the weather is good.

On one particular morning, we skied a few hours, and then suddenly my legs and feet quit responding to my signals to move. There I was, fully outfitted for skiing, with two skis attached to my feet, and two poles in my hands, and I was not going anywhere. I was stuck. My legs were non-responsive and unexplainably fatigued. After a few very long minutes of holding my uncomfortable position on the mountainside so that I would not roll down the ski run as a human snow ball, my neck and back began cramping. My arms were already useless, and I could feel nothing in my toes and fingers. Terrific.

My daughter, who was 8 years-old at the time, knew what had happened to me, and she was as deeply sympathetic as a child can be who is having her fun interrupted. She offered to help me down the mountain so that I would not have to go alone, or worse, let her ski down the mountain by herself. Thus, we turned a routine 10-minute descent down the run into a 45-minute cold and soggy event. When we were half-way down the mountain, my daughter, in an attempt to be helpful and comforting, shouted to me:

"Hey, Mom, you know you could take a Boniva pill for your problem, and your bones would be stronger. You'd only have to take the pill once a month."

I turned my stiff neck to look up the mountain at her and shouted,

"I don't have osteoporosis!"

She shrugged, descended a few more feet, and executed a perfect parallel-ski stop,

"Oh, sorry. I get that confused with what you have. I just thought those old-lady diseases were all the same."

I started sputtering a snappy comeback when she promptly pointed her little skis down the mountain and sped away, well out of earshot. When I caught up with her, she made up for her poorly researched recommendation and caustic jab at my increasing age and decrepitude and, in a true mother-daughter role-reversal she encouraged me to keep going:

"Mom you are looking good. You are doing great. Take it easy. Good job, Mom! You are almost down the hill now!"

She coached me all the way down the mountain in this fashion while skiing in small switch-back patterns to stay with me. When her expert-skier father joined us at the base of the mountain, she broke the magic spell by announcing loudly, "Dad, I need to ski with you, Mom is no fun."

❖ **The Big One**

Fibromyalgia is loosely associated with gastric motility disorders, and the esophagus is part of the gastric anatomy. Thus, scientists speculate that hypersensitivity to pain can predispose a person to abnormal muscular contractions in the gut and throat. In keeping with that kind of craziness, I have esophageal spasms that are literally episodes of excruciating muscle tightening in my throat that extend down toward my stomach. The muscles fire out of harmony, probably due to my body's perception that something is irritating my esophagus, like a too-hot or too-large mouthful of food. Because I am always going somewhere fast, I often quickly eat large bites of food to get it done and move to the next event. So, esophageal spasms are common for me.

When I get esophageal spasms, they are usually so bad that I have to leave the room because I embarrass myself and scare my family—I move my shoulders and neck around and make weird noises as if I am being exorcised of demons. I have learned not to expose others to this bizarre behavior, but I have not always been so smart. The first esophageal spasm I had, I mistook for a heart attack, as the pain is not different from The Big One (think of *Sanford and Son* when Fred clutches his chest and hollers to the Heavens: "I am coming home, Elizabeth, this is The Big One"). If you have ever had an esophageal spasm, you do not need me to explain it. If you have never enjoyed the gripping pain that keeps you from swallowing or breathing, suffice it to say that it is terrifying as it is terrible.

During what I recall as my first esophageal attack, my daughter, who was 3 years-old at the time, was alone with me. The spasm started in my throat, and I felt my neck, face, and chest tighten, and then I couldn't breathe very well. I thought I was going to die. This was particularly terrifying because we had just moved into our new home, in a new city, so we knew no one. During the attack, I could not speak, because I could barely breathe. So, I grabbed the cordless telephone and got into our master bathtub. I took the phone because I thought I might be able to dial 911 before I passed out, and I got into the tub because if I did die, I didn't want my bowels to release and stain our new carpet. Yes, these were the thoughts that were running through my head. I may have been dying, but I wanted to be tidy.

When the spasm passed, after about 8 minutes that felt like an eternity, I was exhausted from fighting the pain, trying to breathe, and keeping calm. I was literally sweating. My daughter found me in the bathtub, still lying there in my sweaty clothing, contemplating things. She gave me a quizzical look, raised one tiny blonde eyebrow, and silently padded out of the bathroom. She seemed to understand—and accept—that I was a little quirky.

❖ Not Enough Sense to Come out of the Rain

Fibromyalgia can make you look crazy. One day in the summer, I walked over to the campus wellness center for my usual lunchtime workout. I noticed that my legs felt heavy during my workout but I braved the treadmill in my traditional way, and I added 15 extra minutes on the elliptical machine to be sure I was not cheating myself out of a good workout simply because I felt a bit "off" that day.

After my exercise, I quickly showered, dressed, and gathered my workout clothes, shoving the whole mess into my gym bag, and I headed out the door...only to find we were in the middle of a downpour, and I had no umbrella. The sky was sunny only one hour before, so I did not anticipate this! I lowered my head and walked out into the rain, thinking I would run back to the office. Interestingly, when I tried to pick up my feet to quicken my pace, my feet would not comply. I was a slow-motion movie compared to the people dashing past me in the rain. When the campus shuttle bus splashed down the street, people peered curiously out the windows at me, as I stared ahead and slowly, robotically slogged through the rain with no umbrella. Their puzzled looks told me all I needed to know: they thought I was insane.

My Exercise Regimen to Control Fibromyalgia

I live better with fibromyalgia when I exercise every day. My exercise routine is not unusual for anyone of my age with general good health, but it might be considered fairly rigorous for someone with fibromyalgia. Nevertheless, I do not think it is unreasonable or unattainable for anyone. Remember that I have had 20 years to become thoroughly fed up with feeling miserable and helpless. That time motivated me to do something about it, on a grand scale, by designing a program for myself.

I am not athletic—not anywhere near it—and, probably like you, I do not have a lot of leisure time. To balance what I need to do for my health against what I am obligated to do as an employee, mother, and wife, I exercise on my lunch hour at work during the week, and I exercise on my own time during the weekend. I recognize that many people do not have this option, and a better idea may be to exercise before or after work. My choices for when I exercise are based on what I can do consistently, with the least amount of disruption for me and my family.

My exercise routine also invites questions from people I know. This often turns into conversations about how busy people are, and ultimately I get the same response: people tell me that they simply do not have time to exercise. When I hear this, I share a trick I learned in Anatomy and Physiology class: consider the time you have in one full day, and make a chart of that day and those activities. On the chart, assign the average time you spend on each task. For example, do you spend one total hour in the car each day as you take children to school and yourself to work, and then, later that day, back home again? If so, then put one hour on the chart for that activity. Do this for all of your daily activities, errands, and chores and then assess the information. Look for 30-minute gaps. Now, ask yourself, "Am I really not able to put 30 minutes or 1 hour of exercise into my day?" I, too, once believed that I had no time to exercise, until I analyzed my actual time spent on tasks over 24 hours. I listed my activities like this:

TABLE 1 ACTIVITIES IN 24 HOURS	
Activity	*Time (hours)*
Sleeping*	6
Working Weekdays	10
Errands	1
Eating meals	2
Driving to work, school, etc.	2
Miscellaneous	3
Total	24.0 hours
*or just lying in the bed, wishing for sleep	

I had to admit, I really had about 3 hours a day filled with nothing at all. Considering the fact that exercise for me only requires about 1/24th of my day—and that my continued good health makes the working, eating, and driving, possible—I should be embarrassed to think that I cannot invest the time. Also, I tell myself that the time will pass at the same rate, whether I am sitting in front of the television or working out, and I have the power to choose how I want to shape that time—for my benefit or for nothing. These thoughts work for me every time.

When I do exercise, I am fairly rigid about my plan, performing 30–50 minutes of cardiovascular exercise and 20 minutes of strength training, plus 5 minutes of stretching or floor exercises. This is my routine for 5 days a week, if time permits, and occasionally I can manage 7 days a week. On the weekends, I can be more flexible with my routine, so I do more low-impact exercises. If I do nothing on the weekend, I am miserable, even with 5 days of working out that week. Thus, daily maintenance for me is best. The table below depicts a sample of a typical week for me:

TABLE 2 WEEKDAY EXERCISE ACTIVITIES	
Monday	
Activity	*Time*
Run on a treadmill	30 minutes
Weight lifting for upper body and arms	20 minutes
Stretching	5 minutes
Stairmaster	15 minutes
Tuesday	
Activity	*Time*
Run on a treadmill	30 minutes
Weight lifting for lower body and legs	20 minutes
Stretching	5 minutes
Stairmaster	15 minutes
Wednesday	
Activity	*Time*
Same as Monday	See above
Thursday	
Activity	*Time*
Same as Tuesday	See above
Friday	
Activity	*Time*
Same as Monday	See above

And here is the weekend:

TABLE 3 WEEKEND EXERCISE ACTIVITIES	
Saturday	
Activity	*Time*
Elliptical Trainer/Swim indoors	45 minutes
Lift weights for total body	25 minutes
Stretch	5 minutes
Sunday	
Activity	*Time*
Run outdoors	55 minutes
Lift weights for total body	25 minutes
Stretch	5 minutes

On the weekend, I prefer easier choices, like the elliptical trainer or running outside, which is always at a slower pace than the treadmill running I do during the week. Because these exercises are lower in intensity, I can exercise longer. This works out well because the weekend is less busy, offering additional time for more exercise.

About twice a month, I simply feel unable to exercise with the necessary vigor and enthusiasm. When my legs and arms feel heavy like this, energetic movement is a little tougher. Thus, on those days, I may begin running at a slower speed and build up to my normal speed, or I might run for fewer minutes on that day. Then, I add something else to my workout to compensate for the diminished activity. I never let myself get away with excuses or giving up. For me, it is easier to go on with the program and do the exercise than to skip it and have to overcome feeling terrible along with resuming exercise after a few days off.

I have a strong mind-set about fibromyalgia. I understand that my body will tell me that I am in pain, but I know that the pain I am feeling is not damaging. I know that the pain I perceive is regulated by a nervous system that oversenses and "overmessages." I am not injured, so I tell myself that have *no excuse* to sit and do nothing. As far as I am concerned, my brain is giving me bad data. So, I override this false information with exercise...which will get me past the faulty signaling and quiet my brain and my body for a short period of time.

This very mental and physical inconsistency often presents extraordinary barriers to exercise in people with fibromyalgia. People do not exercise because they say it "hurts" to exercise. Their brains may be telling them this, but the truth is that exercise will not actually injure them...rather it will make them eventually feel better, if they can overcome this strong signal for a few minutes and do the exercise anyway. Studies to evaluate exercise in people with fibromyalgia often report that simply getting on a program and sticking with it is the greatest obstacle for people with fibromyalgia. However, once someone with fibromyalgia has a few weeks of success, dropping the habit becomes difficult. I have to agree.

When my pain becomes too intense for too many days in a row, I add a yoga class to my exercise routine. Luckily, the wellness center where I exercise at lunchtime has a yoga class once a day, making this easier. The momentary discomfort that I have when beginning the class can be sent to the back of my mind as I focus on the teacher and what we are accomplishing. Also, I know that I will feel better soon, so I practice patience with my yoga poses. If you are intimidated by the thought of trying yoga when you already feel like you cannot move, rest assured that most yoga classes encourage you to work at your own pace. The teachers do not frown upon more slow students, and they are motivated by genuine good will. Thus, they are happy to suggest alternate (easier) postures for the more challenging moves.

My Diet to Control Fibromyalgia

My diet is probably strict, compared to what we are told is the typical American diet, but to me it is fairly generous. This is because my diet serves 4 purposes. First, it gives me the nutrition I need to be present as a mother, wife, and full-time employee, and it fuels my workouts. Next, my diet is an example for my child, modeling what I believe are responsible food choices. Third, my diet enables me to avoid common problems that I encounter with my fibromyalgia, bowel irritability, dizziness, fogginess, and general pain. Finally, my diet keeps me at my desired weight, which helps directly with fibromyalgia in that I am not carrying around extra weight on muscles that are already too tired to handle it. Keeping my weight stable and healthy is good for me indirectly, because it keeps my self-image positive. Honestly, on some days, just looking good trumps feeling good.

My diet evolved over time as I gradually omitted the foods that I could not enjoy without aggravating my fibromyalgia: chocolate; overconsumption of caffeine; fried food; too much of some meats like chicken, turkey, and steak; sugared sodas; and sweets. I am not suggesting that these foods caused my condition and I do not believe that these foods have anything to do with fibromyalgia *per se*. These examples are only specific to me, and they are only presented for general information and curiosity. For example, I have an odd reaction to fried foods: within 15 minutes of eating a piece of fried fish, I am ill and achy, and I just want to lie down...right then. Of course, 15 minutes after my first bite of anything, I am usually still at the table, so I am concerned that I will fall over into my plate in front of my dinner companions. Thus, eliminating these foods is good for me.

You probably deduced that the result of avoiding all of my trigger foods is that my diet is low-sugar, low-fat, and high fiber, abundant in fruits, vegetables, and water. This is more of a happy accident than a plan. *This is simply what I have found works best for me.* I would not suggest that it is desirable for everyone. Your trigger foods, if you have any, may be very different! I also accept that even if my trigger foods are also problematic for others, many of those people will not choose to give up their chocolate or their coffee, because this is too great a sacrifice to make, period. I respect that.

So, mindful of what I need to stay healthy and what I should avoid for my own symptoms, what I eat in a week usually looks like this:

TABLE 4 DAILY DIET

Monday	
Meal	*Food*
Breakfast	2 scrambled eggs, wheat toast, turkey bacon, soy milk, black coffee
Lunch	Spinach salad with 1 c. chopped vegetables, 1 Tbs dressing on the side, fruit, water
Snack	Microwave low-fat popcorn
Dinner	4 oz fish, steamed vegetables, rice or bread, wine
Snack	Apple and peanut butter

Tuesday	
Meal	*Food*
Breakfast	Cereal and soy milk, black coffee, fruit
Lunch	Tuna and 1 Tbs mayonnaise, 10 saltines, fruit, water
Snack	2 pieces of fruit
Dinner	Pasta, seltzer or club soda
Snack	Microwave low-fat popcorn

Wednesday	
Meal	*Food*
Breakfast	Steel-cut oats, 1 package Splenda, ½ c. raw cranberries, black coffee
Lunch	Turkey sandwich on wheat, cucumbers, lettuce, tomato, water
Snack	Apple and peanut butter
Dinner	Rice and beans, seltzer or club soda
Snack	Cut-up fruit with Splenda

Thursday	
Meal	*Food*
Breakfast	Crepes with fruit, black coffee
Lunch	Leftover pasta from home, water
Snack	Fruit
Dinner	Large salad, seltzer or club soda
Snack	Microwave low-fat popcorn

Friday	
Meal	*Food*
Breakfast	Breakfast wrap with eggs and turkey bacon, black coffee, soy milk
Lunch	Soup and salad
Snack	Peanut butter and saltines
Dinner	Sushi, seltzer or club soda
Snack	Pear

The weekend then looks like this:

TABLE 5 DAILY DIET	
Saturday	
Meal	**Food**
Breakfast	Hard boiled egg and 2 pieces wheat toast, black coffee
Lunch	Salad with sliced whole tomato
Snack	Fruit or sugar-free, fat-free yogurt
Dinner	Vegetarian quesadillas, black beans, water
Snack	Microwave low-fat popcorn
Sunday	
Meal	**Food**
Breakfast	Grapefruit, cereal with soy milk, black coffee
Lunch	Salad with lean fish
Snack	Fruit or sugar-free, fat-free yogurt
Dinner	Pasta with vegetables, wine, water
Snack	Tortilla chips and fat-free sour cream

This eating plan is now a way of life for me, after learning to adapt it to fit my fibromyalgia. My meals are purposely small and frequent because I learned that when I eat too much at one sitting, I get esophageal spasms or my IBS takes over, and I sweat, turn red in the face, and need to make an emergency trip to the bathroom. Needless, to say, episodes like that ruin my meal, and they are not worth inviting again. Necessity may be the Mother of Invention, but I will swear that Desperation is the Father of Drastic Change.

If you must go out for dinner due to work or other obligations, meals may present a significant challenge for you. My family does not go out to dinner much more than once a month because I can cook more cheaply and healthfully, and I feel better when I know what goes into what I am eating. Also, my family enjoys meal times together because we can talk while I cook and we continue our conversation over dinner and beyond. On the occasion that I do go out to dinner, I have found that a salad with a dressing on the side, a simple pasta dish, or baked fish with steamed vegetables is usually available. That kind of meal, accompanied by lots of water with lemon, is satisfactory. If certain foods make you feel lousy and restaurants are difficult for you, too, you may want to experiment with options that please your palate as well as keep your flare-ups under control.

I hope that you do not look at my approach and immediately think: well, this is hopeless: I just cannot do that. Don't worry. Ideally, my routine may just give you some ideas of what to do for yourself. My routine evolved over 20 years of trying something new almost monthly and then eliminating what was not helpful. I am sure you appreciate that changing something takes a lot of discipline, and often that discipline is too difficult to call on when you feel terrible. That is ok. Experiment and be inventive. If you do have a success, reward yourself. This will motivate you to try something new again.

Life Changes I Make for Fibromyalgia

As you already know, fibromyalgia ruins sleep. The cycle of not being able to sleep because of your pain, coupled with needing sleep to make the pain go away, is vicious. On days that follow nights when I do not get enough sleep, I know that I should change my routine to be safe. For example, the day after a night of no sleep is a day in which I am very cautious about taking risks with me or my family, such as when driving the car to work or taking my child to school. I look twice before passing through an intersection, and I limit my driving trips around town that day. Also, on days when I am foggy and sleepy, I try to limit any lasting or critical decisions until I have had rest.

When I do enjoy the luxury of a few hours of uninterrupted sleep, my fibromyalgia wakes me up like an alarm clock before the sun rises in the morning. My legs and back scream with pain and I am wide awake. From these episodes, I have learned that I cannot be still for too long. This applies to sleeping, sitting, and standing and any activity that requires me to do those things for a long time. Being in a car too long aggravates my fibromyalgia. Similar confinement such as flying in an airplane, stuck in a tiny seat, for many hours will drive me crazy to the point that I actively limit my flying overseas, much to the disappointment of my family. Sitting for hours at work makes me uncomfortable, so I get up every hour and walk around my office, get a glass of water from the cooler, or take a bathroom break.

Binding or tight clothing can worsen my fibromyalgia pain, so I must deliberately choose clothes that are loose in the shoulders or waist. Likewise, clothes that rub and chafe can make me miserable because I am highly sensitive to any potentially painful stimulus. I also keep my jewelry simple and to a minimum. For example, I avoid heavy necklaces, which aggravate my neck pain. High-heel shoes are fine now and then, but I try to rotate my shoes to prevent my feet, legs, and lower back from cramping and giving me grief for the rest of the day.

Around the house, I have inexpensive devices to make cooking and cleaning more manageable. I have a great can opener, an easy wine-cork puller, and lots of plastic tools that don't break when I drop them. Also, I use a folded beach towel under my knees when I must kneel on the ground to garden or clean something. This helps with the grinding pain that comes from putting weight on my knees. Also, textured gloves help me grip weeds or tools when I work in the yard and they protect my hands. If you give it thought, and you are willing to experiment, you can improve your comfort while undertaking almost any chore.

Tackling Bad Episodes

When I have a particularly bad episode of fibromyalgia, if I happen to be at home, I will lie on the floor and stretch for a few minutes, targeting what specifically bothers me. I *force* myself to do this, becoming angry at my pain and at myself for being lazy and not wanting to do anything about it. Usually, after about five minutes of really intense stretching, I feel a little more sane, and the more exercise I do, the better I feel. As you know, it takes an enormous energy of activation (energy just to get something *started*) to actually do something to manage fibromyalgia when it is bad. However, I understand that I can control much of what I experience. As you can probably tell, I actively handle my fibromyalgia and I do very few passive activities. To me, active participation means active control. This is partly due to my personality of wanting to be in charge of my health and partly due to bad experiences with passively managing my pain with medications in the past.

Although I describe a host of medications in Chapter 4, which is dedicated to drug therapies for fibromyalgia, and there are presently 3 new drugs approved for this condition, I elect not to use drug therapy to manage my situation. That may sound unreasonable, to have a solution and then to walk away from it. My rationale is simple: I would rather manage it on my own without the need for drugs that I may not always have access to or the money to buy. I figure that by having real solutions for my fibromyalgia that are ultimately in my hands, I am doing more for myself than any drug could. This approach is not suitable for everyone. I offer the information to give those who cannot purchase medications or obtain prescriptions for these drugs reasonable options for non-drug ideas.

Interestingly, over time, I have recognized that many drugs do not work well for me. For example, I learned the hard way that I cannot take opioids or opiates (narcotics), so many prescription pain medications are useless for my pain or just harmful for me. People with fibromyalgia are reported to have increased drug side effects,[64, 65] but because of past experiences with medications, I do not think this is the cause for *my* particular drug sensitivities. Rather, my sensitivity to narcotics is due to an inability of my body to break down or effectively metabolize a certain class of drugs that follow a specific metabolic pathway in the liver. Evidence for this comes from the fact that I have the same reactions to every drug in this class, and the fact that my family members have similar reactions. I also know from my science background that genetic differences in the way our bodies handle medications can have significant implications in what therapies work best for us. So, instead of pain relief from drugs that are very helpful to other people, I get histamine release (causes itching) agitation, depersonalization (feeling like I am out of my body), and limb jerking. Drug side effects like these are worth noting, and people who experience similar issues should investigate new medications with care.

Final Words

Fibromyalgia is a burden that can decrease anyone's quality of life.[414] Thus, because of the unique symptoms—fatigue, intolerance to exercise and exertion, headaches, etc, it is very easy to refuse to do anything about it and to instead accept a life that is less than full and to adopt a demeanor that is less than enthusiastic and positive. I understand this too well, and I am often under the spell of the fibromyalgia monster, more willing to write off another precious day to self-misery than to turn my day around with a few minutes of effort. The bottom line is that I cannot die from my fibromyalgia, I can only be inconvenienced by it, and that is just not a sufficient reason to do nothing about it! So, I wish for you what I wish for myself: a today better than yesterday and a tomorrow that excites you with the promise of what it will bring.

INDEX

D

E

F

S

T

BIBLIOGRAPHY

1. Chakrabarty S, Zoorob R. Fibromyalgia. Am Fam Physician 2007;76(2):247-54.

2. Pamuk ON, Yesil Y, Cakir N. Factors that affect the number of tender points in fibromyalgia and chronic widespread pain patients who did not meet the ACR 1990 criteria for fibromyalgia: are tender points a reflection of neuropathic pain? Semin Arthritis Rheum 2006;36(2):130-4.

3. Russell IJ, Raphael KG. Fibromyalgia syndrome: presentation, diagnosis, differential diagnosis, and vulnerability. CNS Spectr 2008;13(3 Suppl 5):6-11.

4. Wolfe F. Fibromyalgia. Rheum Dis Clin North Am 1990;16(3):681-98.

5. Wolfe F, Smythe HA, Yunus MB, Bennett RM, Bombardier C, Goldenberg DL, Tugwell P, Campbell SM, Abeles M, Clark P, et al. The American College of Rheumatology 1990 Criteria for the Classification of Fibromyalgia. Report of the Multicenter Criteria Committee. Arthritis Rheum 1990;33(2):160-72.

6. Wolfe F. The clinical syndrome of fibrositis. Am J Med 1986;81(3A):7-14.

7. Clauw DJ. Fibromyalgia: more than just a musculoskeletal disease. Am Fam Physician 1995;52(3):843-51, 53-4.

8. Huynh CN, Yanni LM, Morgan LA. Key practice points in the management of fibromyalgia. Am Fam Physician 2007;76(2):195-6, 202.

9. Moldofsky H. The significance, assessment, and management of nonrestorative sleep in fibromyalgia syndrome. CNS Spectr 2008;13(3 Suppl 5):22-6.

10. Togo F, Natelson BH, Cherniack NS, Fitzgibbons J, Garcon C, Rapoport DM. Sleep structure and sleepiness in chronic fatigue syndrome with or without coexisting fibromyalgia. Arthritis Res Ther 2008;10(3):R56.

11. Shaver JL, Lentz M, Landis CA, Heitkemper MM, Buchwald DS, Woods NF. Sleep, psychological distress, and stress arousal in women with fibromyalgia. Res Nurs Health 1997;20(3):247-57.

12. Burns JW, Crofford LJ, Chervin RD. Sleep stage dynamics in fibromyalgia patients and controls. Sleep Med 2008.

13. Reiter RJ, Acuna-Castroviejo D, Tan DX. Melatonin therapy in fibromyalgia. Curr Pain Headache Rep 2007;11(5):339-42.

14. Davis GC. Improved sleep may reduce arthritis pain. Holist Nurs Pract 2003;17(3):128-35.

15. Drewes AM, Nielsen KD, Arendt-Nielsen L, Birket-Smith L, Hansen LM. The effect of cutaneous and deep pain on the electroencephalogram during sleep--an experimental study. Sleep 1997;20(8):632-40.

16. Kundermann B, Krieg JC, Schreiber W, Lautenbacher S. The effect of sleep deprivation on pain. Pain Res Manag 2004;9(1):25-32.

17. Mahowald ML, Mahowald MW. Nighttime sleep and daytime functioning (sleepiness and fatigue) in less well-defined chronic rheumatic diseases with particular reference to the 'alpha-delta NREM sleep anomaly'. Sleep Med 2000;1(3):195-207.

18. Jones KD, Clark SR, Bennett RM. Prescribing exercise for people with fibromyalgia. AACN Clin Issues 2002;13(2):277-93.

19. Klerman EB, Goldenberg DL, Brown EN, Maliszewski AM, Adler GK. Circadian rhythms of women with fibromyalgia. J Clin Endocrinol Metab 2001;86(3):1034-9.

20. Sarzi-Puttini P, Rizzi M, Andreoli A, Panni B, Pecis M, Colombo S, Turiel M, Carrabba M, Sergi M. Hypersomnolence in fibromyalgia syndrome. Clin Exp Rheumatol 2002;20(1):69-72.

21. Menefee LA, Cohen MJ, Anderson WR, Doghramji K, Frank ED, Lee H. Sleep disturbance and nonmalignant chronic pain: a comprehensive review of the literature. Pain Med 2000;1(2):156-72.

22. Wikner J, Hirsch U, Wetterberg L, Rojdmark S. Fibromyalgia--a syndrome associated with decreased nocturnal melatonin secretion. Clin Endocrinol (Oxf) 1998;49(2):179-83.

23. Moldofsky H, Scarisbrick P, England R, Smythe H. Musculosketal symptoms and non-REM sleep disturbance in patients with "fibrositis syndrome" and healthy subjects. Psychosom Med 1975;37(4):341-51.

24. Juhl JH. Fibromyalgia and the serotonin pathway. Altern Med Rev 1998;3(5):367-75.

25. Perez-Ruiz F, Calabozo M, Alonso-Ruiz A, Ruiz-Lucea E. Fibromyalgia and carpal tunnel syndrome. Ann Rheum Dis 1997;56(7):438-9.

26. Nielsen LA, Henriksson KG. Pathophysiological mechanisms in chronic musculoskeletal pain (fibromyalgia): the role of central and peripheral sensitization and pain disinhibition. Best Pract Res Clin Rheumatol 2007;21(3):465-80.

27. Nielens H, Boisset V, Masquelier E. Fitness and perceived exertion in patients with fibromyalgia syndrome. Clin J Pain 2000;16(3):209-13.

28. Staud R. Future perspectives: pathogenesis of chronic muscle pain. Best Pract Res Clin Rheumatol 2007;21(3):581-96.

29. Arnold LM. Biology and therapy of fibromyalgia. New therapies in fibromyalgia. Arthritis Res Ther 2006;8(4):212.

30. Thompson D, Lettich L, Takeshita J. Fibromyalgia: an overview. Curr Psychiatry Rep 2003;5(3):211-7.

31. Miller LJ, Kubes KL. Serotonergic agents in the treatment of fibromyalgia syndrome. Ann Pharmacother 2002;36(4):707-12.

32. Abeles AM, Pillinger MH, Solitar BM, Abeles M. Narrative review: the pathophysiology of fibromyalgia. Ann Intern Med 2007;146(10):726-34.

33. Schweinhardt P, Sauro KM, Bushnell MC. Fibromyalgia: A Disorder of the Brain? Neuroscientist 2008.

34. Vaeroy H, Qiao ZG, Morkrid L, Forre O. Altered sympathetic nervous system response in patients with fibromyalgia (fibrositis syndrome). J Rheumatol 1989;16(11):1460-5.

35. Bennett RM, Clark SR, Campbell SM, Ingram SB, Burckhardt CS, Nelson DL, Porter JM. Symptoms of Raynaud's syndrome in patients with fibromyalgia. A study utilizing the Nielsen test, digital photoplethysmography, and measurements of platelet alpha 2-adrenergic receptors. Arthritis Rheum 1991;34(3):264-9.

36. Chial HJ, Camilleri M. Gender differences in irritable bowel syndrome. J Gend Specif Med 2002;5(3):37-45.

37. Kurland JE, Coyle WJ, Winkler A, Zable E. Prevalence of irritable bowel syndrome and depression in fibromyalgia. Dig Dis Sci 2006;51(3):454-60.

38. Kwan CL, Diamant NE, Pope G, Mikula K, Mikulis DJ, Davis KD. Abnormal forebrain activity in functional bowel disorder patients with chronic pain. Neurology 2005;65(8):1268-77.

39. Mayer EA, Fass R, Fullerton S. Intestinal and extraintestinal symptoms in functional gastrointestinal disorders. Eur J Surg Suppl 1998(583):29-31.

40. Triadafilopoulos G, Simms RW, Goldenberg DL. Bowel dysfunction in fibromyalgia syndrome. Dig Dis Sci 1991;36(1):59-64.

41. Veale D, Kavanagh G, Fielding JF, Fitzgerald O. Primary fibromyalgia and the irritable bowel syndrome: different expressions of a common pathogenetic process. Br J Rheumatol 1991;30(3):220-2.

42. Verne GN, Price DD. Irritable bowel syndrome as a common precipitant of central sensitization. Curr Rheumatol Rep 2002;4(4):322-8.

43. Wallace DJ, Hallegua DS. Fibromyalgia: the gastrointestinal link. Curr Pain Headache Rep 2004;8(5):364-8.

44. Chang L. The association of functional gastrointestinal disorders and fibromyalgia. Eur J Surg Suppl 1998(583):32-6.

45. Klevmark B. [Frequent urination]. Tidsskr Nor Laegeforen 2005;125(5):624-5; author reply 5.

46. Talseth T, Hedlund H. [Frequent urination and fibromyalgia]. Tidsskr Nor Laegeforen 2005;125(5):623-4; author reply 4.

47. Stormorken H, Brosstad F. [Frequent urination--an important diagnostic marker in fibromyalgia]. Tidsskr Nor Laegeforen 2005;125(1):17-9.

48. Wyller TB, Wyller VB. [Fibromyalgia, urination and established truths]. Tidsskr Nor Laegeforen 2005;125(1):14.

49. Wallace DJ. Genitourinary manifestations of fibrositis: an increased association with the female urethral syndrome. J Rheumatol 1990;17(2):238-9.

50. Brand K, Littlejohn G, Kristjanson L, Wisniewski S, Hassard T. The fibromyalgia bladder index. Clin Rheumatol 2007;26(12):2097-103.

51. Schuh-Hofer S, Richter M, Geworski L, Villringer A, Israel H, Wenzel R, Munz DL, Arnold G. Increased serotonin transporter availability in the brainstem of migraineurs. J Neurol 2007;254(6):789-96.

52. Nicolodi M, Volpe AR, Sicuteri F. Fibromyalgia and headache. Failure of serotonergic analgesia and N-methyl-D-aspartate-mediated neuronal plasticity: their common clues. Cephalalgia 1998;18 Suppl 21:41-4.

53. Peres MF, Young WB, Kaup AO, Zukerman E, Silberstein SD. Fibromyalgia is common in patients with transformed migraine. Neurology 2001;57(7):1326-8.

54. Kaiser RS. "Raynaud's disease" in migraineurs: one entity or two? Headache 1992;32(9):463-5.

55. Hudson JI, Goldenberg DL, Pope HG, Jr., Keck PE, Jr., Schlesinger L. Comorbidity of fibromyalgia with medical and psychiatric disorders. Am J Med 1992;92(4):363-7.

56. Guler M, Kirnap M, Bekaroglu M, Uremek G, Onder C. Clinical characteristics of patients with fibromyalgia. Isr J Med Sci 1992;28(1):20-3.

57. Sarmer S, Yavuzer G, Kucukdeveci A, Ergin S. Prevalence of carpal tunnel syndrome in patients with fibromyalgia. Rheumatol Int 2002;22(2):68-70.

58. Martinez-Lavin M, Lopez S, Medina M, Nava A. Use of the leeds assessment of neuropathic symptoms and signs questionnaire in patients with fibromyalgia. Semin Arthritis Rheum 2003;32(6):407-11.

59. Caro XJ, Winter EF, Dumas AJ. A subset of fibromyalgia patients have findings suggestive of chronic inflammatory demyelinating polyneuropathy and appear to respond to IVIg. Rheumatology [Oxford] 2008;47(2):208-11.

60. Ersoz M. Nerve conduction tests in patients with fibromyalgia: comparison with normal controls. Rheumatol Int 2003;23(4):166-70.

61. Moshiree B, Price DD, Robinson ME, Gaible R, Verne GN. Thermal and visceral hypersensitivity in irritable bowel syndrome patients with and without fibromyalgia. Clin J Pain 2007;23(4):323-30.

62. Geisser ME, Casey KL, Brucksch CB, Ribbens CM, Appleton BB, Crofford LJ. Perception of noxious and innocuous heat stimulation among healthy women and women with fibromyalgia: association with mood, somatic focus, and catastrophizing. Pain 2003;102(3):243-50.

63. Berglund B, Harju EL, Kosek E, Lindblom U. Quantitative and qualitative perceptual analysis of cold dysesthesia and hyperalgesia in fibromyalgia. Pain 2002;96(1-2):177-87.

64. Skeith KJ, Hussain MS, Coutts RT, Ramos-Remus C, Avina-Zubieta JA, Russell AS. Adverse drug reactions and debrisoquine/sparteine (P450IID6) polymorphism in patients with fibromyalgia. Clin Rheumatol 1997;16(3):291-5.

65. Rico-Villademoros F, Hidalgo J, Dominguez I, Garcia-Leiva JM, Calandre EP. Atypical antipsychotics in the treatment of fibromyalgia: a case series with olanzapine. Prog Neuropsychopharmacol Biol Psychiatry 2005;29(1):161-4.

66. Holtedahl R. [Analgesics use in patients with chronic musculoskeletal complaints]. Tidsskr Nor Laegeforen 2004;124(15):1930-2.

67. Markowitz J, Patrick K. Polypharmacy side effects. J Am Acad Child Adolesc Psychiatry 1996;35(7):842.

68. Akici A, Oktay S. Rational pharmacotherapy and pharmacovigilance. Curr Drug Saf 2007;2(1):65-9.

69. Graham W. Fibrositis and non-articular rheumatism. Phys Ther Rev 1955;35(3):128-33.

70. [No authors listed]. Arthritis & other rheumatic disorders. II. Non-articular rheumatism and fibrositis. Q Med Rev 1971;22(1):1-20.

71. Holbrook WP. Soft tissue rheumatism. Gp 1952;6(5):53-9.

72. Svartz N. Is "muscular rheumatism" a rheumatic disease? Acta Med Scand Suppl 1952;266:915-7.

73. Graham W. Fibrositis and non-articular rheumatism. Physiotherapy 1954;40(4):101-4.

74. Crowe HW. Preliminary report: trafuril in the treatment of muscular rheumatism. Rheumatism 1951;7(4):75-7.

75. Laughton-Scott G. Rheumatic fibrositis--some speculations. Med World 1952;76(1):8-10.

76. Martin AJ. The nature and treatment of fibrositis. Arch Phys Med Rehabil 1952;33(7):409-13.

77. Warter PJ. Soft tissue distress in rheumatic disease. J Med Soc N J 1956;53(8):407-11.

78. Callahan LF, Pincus T. A clue from a self-report questionnaire to distinguish rheumatoid arthritis from noninflammatory diffuse musculoskeletal pain. The P-VAS:D-ADL ratio. Arthritis Rheum 1990;33(9):1317-22.

79. Staud R, Smitherman ML. Peripheral and central sensitization in fibromyalgia: pathogenetic role. Curr Pain Headache Rep 2002;6(4):259-66.

80. Jacobsen S, Bredkjaer SR. The prevalence of fibromyalgia and widespread chronic musculoskeletal pain in the general population. Scand J Rheumatol 1992;21(5):261-3.

81. Wolfe F, Ross K, Anderson J, Russell IJ, Hebert L. The prevalence and characteristics of fibromyalgia in the general population. Arthritis Rheum 1995;38(1):19-28.

82. Peterson EL. Fibromyalgia--management of a misunderstood disorder. J Am Acad Nurse Pract 2007;19(7):341-8.

83. Rao SG, Gendreau JF, Kranzler JD. Understanding the fibromyalgia syndrome. Psychopharmacol Bull 2007;40(4):24-67.

84. Makela M, Heliovaara M. Prevalence of primary fibromyalgia in the Finnish population. Bmj 1991;303(6796):216-9.

85. Forseth KO, Gran JT. The prevalence of fibromyalgia among women aged 20-49 years in Arendal, Norway. Scand J Rheumatol 1992;21(2):74-8.

86. Weir PT, Harlan GA, Nkoy FL, Jones SS, Hegmann KT, Gren LH, Lyon JL. The incidence of fibromyalgia and its associated comorbidities: a population-based retrospective cohort study based on International Classification of Diseases, 9th Revision codes. J Clin Rheumatol 2006;12(3):124-8.

87. Buskila D, Neumann L, Hazanov I, Carmi R. Familial aggregation in the fibromyalgia syndrome. Semin Arthritis Rheum 1996;26(3):605-11.

88. Buskila D, Press J, Gedalia A, Klein M, Neumann L, Boehm R, Sukenik S. Assessment of nonarticular tenderness and prevalence of fibromyalgia in children. J Rheumatol 1993;20(2):368-70.

89. Eraso RM, Bradford NJ, Fontenot CN, Espinoza LR, Gedalia A. Fibromyalgia syndrome in young children: onset at age 10 years and younger. Clin Exp Rheumatol 2007;25(4):639-44.

90. Anthony KK, Schanberg LE. Juvenile primary fibromyalgia syndrome. Curr Rheumatol Rep 2001;3(2):165-71.

91. Degotardi PJ, Klass ES, Rosenberg BS, Fox DG, Gallelli KA, Gottlieb BS. Development and evaluation of a cognitive-behavioral intervention for juvenile fibromyalgia. J Pediatr Psychol 2006;31(7):714-23.

92. Buskila D, Neumann L, Hershman E, Gedalia A, Press J, Sukenik S. Fibromyalgia syndrome in children--an outcome study. J Rheumatol 1995;22(3):525-8.

93. Buskila D, Neumann L, Press J. Genetic factors in neuromuscular pain. CNS Spectr 2005;10(4):281-4.

94. Neumann L, Buskila D. Epidemiology of fibromyalgia. Curr Pain Headache Rep 2003;7(5):362-8.

95. Stormorken H, Brosstad F. Fibromyalgia: family clustering and sensory urgency with early onset indicate genetic predisposition and thus a "true" disease. Scand J Rheumatol 1992;21(4):207.

96. Pellegrino MJ, Waylonis GW, Sommer A. Familial occurrence of primary fibromyalgia. Arch Phys Med Rehabil 1989;70(1):61-3.

97. Weissbecker I, Floyd A, Dedert E, Salmon P, Sephton S. Childhood trauma and diurnal cortisol disruption in fibromyalgia syndrome. Psychoneuroendocrinology 2006;31(3):312-24.

98. Buskila D. Genetics of chronic pain states. Best Pract Res Clin Rheumatol 2007;21(3):535-47.

99. Van Houdenhove B, Egle U, Luyten P. The role of life stress in fibromyalgia. Curr Rheumatol Rep 2005;7(5):365-70.

100. Boscarino JA. Posttraumatic stress disorder and physical illness: results from clinical and epidemiologic studies. Ann N Y Acad Sci 2004;1032:141-53.

101. Ablin JN, Shoenfeld Y, Buskila D. Fibromyalgia, infection and vaccination: Two more parts in the etiological puzzle. J Autoimmun 2006;27(3):145-52.

102. Nasralla M, Haier J, Nicolson GL. Multiple mycoplasmal infections detected in blood of patients with chronic fatigue syndrome and/or fibromyalgia syndrome. Eur J Clin Microbiol Infect Dis 1999;18(12):859-65.

103. Ribeiro LS, Proietti FA. Interrelations between fibromyalgia, thyroid autoantibodies, and depression. J Rheumatol 2004;31(10):2036-40.

104. Staines DR. Is fibromyalgia an autoimmune disorder of endogenous vasoactive neuropeptides? Med Hypotheses 2004;62(5):665-9.

105. Frieri M. Identification of masqueraders of autoimmune disease in the office. Allergy Asthma Proc 2003;24(6):421-9.

106. Littlejohn GO, Weinstein C, Helme RD. Increased neurogenic inflammation in fibrositis syndrome. J Rheumatol 1987;14(5):1022-5.

107. McDermid AJ, Rollman GB, McCain GA. Generalized hypervigilance in fibromyalgia: evidence of perceptual amplification. Pain 1996;66(2-3):133-44.

108. Crombez G, Eccleston C, Van den Broeck A, Goubert L, Van Houdenhove B. Hypervigilance to pain in fibromyalgia: the mediating role of pain intensity and catastrophic thinking about pain. Clin J Pain 2004;20(2):98-102.

109. Rollman GB. Measurement of pain in fibromyalgia in the clinic and laboratory. J Rheumatol Suppl 1989;19:113-9.

110. Staud R, Spaeth M. Psychophysical and neurochemical abnormalities of pain processing in fibromyalgia. CNS Spectr 2008;13(3 Suppl 5):12-7.

111. Kotter I, Neuscheler D, Gunaydin I, Wernet D, Klein R. Is there a predisposition for the development of autoimmune diseases in patients with fibromyalgia? Retrospective analysis with long term follow-up. Rheumatol Int 2007;27(11):1031-9.

112. Jacobsen S, Hoyer-Madsen M, Danneskiold-Samsoe B, Wiik A. Screening for autoantibodies in patients with primary fibromyalgia syndrome and a matched control group. Apmis 1990;98(7):655-8.

113. Steiner G. Auto-antibodies and autoreactive T-cells in rheumatoid arthritis: pathogenetic players and diagnostic tools. Clin Rev Allergy Immunol 2007;32(1):23-36.

114. Schwendimann RN, Alekseeva N. Gender issues in multiple sclerosis. Int Rev Neurobiol 2007;79:377-92.

115. Kerns RD, Kassirer M, Otis J. Pain in multiple sclerosis: a biopsychosocial perspective. J Rehabil Res Dev 2002;39(2):225-32.

116. Howarth AL. Pain management for multiple sclerosis patients. Prof Nurse 2000;16(1):824-6.

117. Belogurov AA, Jr., Kurkova IN, Friboulet A, Thomas D, Misikov VK, Zakharova MY, Suchkov SV, Kotov SV, Alehin AI, Avalle B, Souslova EA, Morse HC, 3rd, Gabibov AG, Ponomarenko NA. Recognition and degradation of myelin basic protein peptides by serum autoantibodies: novel biomarker for multiple sclerosis. J Immunol 2008;180(2):1258-67.

118. Hellings N, Baree M, Verhoeven C, D'Hooghe M B, Medaer R, Bernard CC, Raus J, Stinissen P. T-cell reactivity to multiple myelin antigens in multiple sclerosis patients and healthy controls. J Neurosci Res 2001;63(3):290-302.

119. Sinaii N, Cleary SD, Ballweg ML, Nieman LK, Stratton P. High rates of autoimmune and endocrine disorders, fibromyalgia, chronic fatigue syndrome and atopic diseases among women with endometriosis: a survey analysis. Hum Reprod 2002;17(10):2715-24.

120. Staud R. Are patients with systemic lupus erythematosus at increased risk for fibromyalgia? Curr Rheumatol Rep 2006;8(6):430-5.

121. Moldovan I. Systemic lupus erythematosus: current state of diagnosis and treatment. Compr Ther 2006;32(3):158-62.

122. Lockshin MD. Sex differences in autoimmune disease. Lupus 2006;15(11):753-6.

123. Bengtsson A, Ernerudh J, Vrethem M, Skogh T. Absence of autoantibodies in primary fibromyalgia. J Rheumatol 1990;17(12):1682-3.

124. Ulvestad E. Modelling autoimmune rheumatic disease: a likelihood rationale. Scand J Immunol 2003;58(1):106-11.

125. Kim SH. Skin biopsy findings: implications for the pathophysiology of fibromyalgia. Med Hypotheses 2007;69(1):141-4.

126. Kim SH, Jang TJ, Moon IS. Increased expression of N-methyl-D-aspartate receptor subunit 2D in the skin of patients with fibromyalgia. J Rheumatol 2006;33(4):785-8.

127. Kim SH, Kim DH, Oh DH, Clauw DJ. Characteristic electron microscopic findings in the skin of patients with fibromyalgia--preliminary study. Clin Rheumatol 2008;27(3):407-11.

128. Bengtsson A, Henriksson KG, Larsson J. Muscle biopsy in primary fibromyalgia. Light-microscopical and histochemical findings. Scand J Rheumatol 1986;15(1):1-6.

129. Yunus MB, Kalyan-Raman UP, Kalyan-Raman K, Masi AT. Pathologic changes in muscle in primary fibromyalgia syndrome. Am J Med 1986;81(3A):38-42.

130. Elam M, Johansson G, Wallin BG. Do patients with primary fibromyalgia have an altered muscle sympathetic nerve activity? Pain 1992;48(3):371-5.

131. Kivimaki M, Leino-Arjas P, Virtanen M, Elovainio M, Keltikangas-Jarvinen L, Puttonen S, Vartia M, Brunner E, Vahtera J. Work stress and incidence of newly diagnosed fibromyalgia: prospective cohort study. J Psychosom Res 2004;57(5):417-22.

132. Shanklin DR, Stevens MV, Hall MF, Smalley DL. Environmental immunogens and T-cell-mediated responses in fibromyalgia: evidence for immune dysregulation and determinants of granuloma formation. Exp Mol Pathol 2000;69(2):102-18.

133. Bell IR, Baldwin CM, Schwartz GE. Illness from low levels of environmental chemicals: relevance to chronic fatigue syndrome and fibromyalgia. Am J Med 1998;105(3A):74S-82S.

134. Banic B, Petersen-Felix S, Andersen OK, Radanov BP, Villiger PM, Arendt-Nielsen L, Curatolo M. Evidence for spinal cord hypersensitivity in chronic pain after whiplash injury and in fibromyalgia. Pain 2004;107(1-2):7-15.

135. Ferrari R, Shorter E. From railway spine to whiplash--the recycling of nervous irritation. Med Sci Monit 2003;9(11):HY27-37.

136. Hoppmann RA. Instrumental musicians' hazards. Occup Med 2001;16(4):619-31, iv-v.

137. Pinals RS. Nonarticular rheumatism, sports-related injuries, and related conditions. Curr Opin Rheumatol 1997;9(2):133-4.

138. Ablin J, Neumann L, Buskila D. Pathogenesis of fibromyalgia - a review. Joint Bone Spine 2008;75(3):273-9.

139. Poyhia R, Da Costa D, Fitzcharles MA. Previous pain experience in women with fibromyalgia and inflammatory arthritis and nonpainful controls. J Rheumatol 2001;28(8):1888-91.

140. Goldberg RT, Pachas WN, Keith D. Relationship between traumatic events in childhood and chronic pain. Disabil Rehabil 1999;21(1):23-30.

141. Keel P. Psychological and psychiatric aspects of fibromyalgia syndrome (FMS). Z Rheumatol 1998;57 Suppl 2:97-100.

142. Bell IR, Baldwin CM, Russek LG, Schwartz GE, Hardin EE. Early life stress, negative paternal relationships, and chemical intolerance in middle-aged women: support for a neural sensitization model. J Womens Health 1998;7(9):1135-47.

143. Amir M, Kaplan Z, Neumann L, Sharabani R, Shani N, Buskila D. Posttraumatic stress disorder, tenderness and fibromyalgia. J Psychosom Res 1997;42(6):607-13.

144. Tishler M, Levy O, Maslakov I, Bar-Chaim S, Amit-Vazina M. Neck injury and fibromyalgia— are they really associated? J Rheumatol 2006;33(6):1183-5.

145. Conte PM, Walco GA, Kimura Y. Temperament and stress response in children with juvenile primary fibromyalgia syndrome. Arthritis Rheum 2003;48(10):2923-30.

146. Gur A, Oktayoglu P. Central nervous system abnormalities in fibromyalgia and chronic fatigue syndrome: new concepts in treatment. Curr Pharm Des 2008;14(13):1274-94.

147. McCabe CS, Cohen H, Blake DR. Somaesthetic disturbances in fibromyalgia are exaggerated by sensory motor conflict: implications for chronicity of the disease? Rheumatology (Oxford) 2007;46(10):1587-92.

148. Sitges C, Garcia-Herrera M, Pericas M, Collado D, Truyols M, Montoya P. Abnormal brain processing of affective and sensory pain descriptors in chronic pain patients. J Affect Disord 2007;104(1-3):73-82.

149. Martinez-Lavin M. Fibromyalgia as a sympathetically maintained pain syndrome. Curr Pain Headache Rep 2004;8(5):385-9.

150. Crofford LJ, Engleberg NC, Demitrack MA. Neurohormonal perturbations in fibromyalgia. Baillieres Clin Rheumatol 1996;10(2):365-78.

151. Dohrenbusch R. [Are patients with fibromyalgia "hypervigilant"?]. Schmerz 2001;15(1):38-47.

152. Staud R, Domingo M. Evidence for abnormal pain processing in fibromyalgia syndrome. Pain Med 2001;2(3):208-15.

153. Wolff HG, Hardy JD, Goodell H. Experimental studies on the nature of hyperalgesia. Arch Neurol Psychiatry 1950;63(1):188.

154. Sorensen J, Graven-Nielsen T, Henriksson KG, Bengtsson M, Arendt-Nielsen L. Hyperexcitability in fibromyalgia. J Rheumatol 1998;25(1):152-5.

155. Arroyo JF, Cohen ML. Abnormal responses to electrocutaneous stimulation in fibromyalgia. J Rheumatol 1993;20(11):1925-31.

156. Henriksson KG. Hypersensitivity in muscle pain syndromes. Curr Pain Headache Rep 2003;7(6):426-32.

157. Le Page JA, Iverson GL, Collins P. The impact of judges' perceptions of credibility in fibromyalgia claims. Int J Law Psychiatry 2008;31(1):30-40.

158. Asbring P, Narvanen AL. Ideal versus reality: physicians perspectives on patients with chronic fatigue syndrome (CFS) and fibromyalgia. Soc Sci Med 2003;57(4):711-20.

159. Vargas A, Vargas A, Hernandez-Paz R, Sanchez-Huerta JM, Romero-Ramirez R, Amezcua-Guerra L, Kooh M, Nava A, Pineda C, Rodriguez-Leal G, Martinez-Lavin M. Sphygmomanometry-evoked allodynia--a simple bedside test indicative of fibromyalgia: a multicenter developmental study. J Clin Rheumatol 2006;12(6):272-4.

160. Ottley C. Food and mood. Nurs Stand 2000;15(2):46-52; quiz 4-5.

161. Benton D, Donohoe RT. The effects of nutrients on mood. Public Health Nutr 1999;2(3A):403-9.

162. Bruinsma K, Taren DL. Chocolate: food or drug? J Am Diet Assoc 1999;99(10):1249-56.

163. Moller SE. Serotonin, carbohydrates, and atypical depression. Pharmacol Toxicol 1992;71 Suppl 1:61-71.

164. Wood PB. Role of central dopamine in pain and analgesia. Expert Rev Neurother 2008;8(5):781-97.

165. Wood PB, Patterson JC, 2nd, Sunderland JJ, Tainter KH, Glabus MF, Lilien DL. Reduced presynaptic dopamine activity in fibromyalgia syndrome demonstrated with positron emission tomography: a pilot study. J Pain 2007;8(1):51-8.

166. Wood PB. Stress and dopamine: implications for the pathophysiology of chronic widespread pain. Med Hypotheses 2004;62(3):420-4.

167. Malt EA, Olafsson S, Aakvaag A, Lund A, Ursin H. Altered dopamine D2 receptor function in fibromyalgia patients: a neuroendocrine study with buspirone in women with fibromyalgia compared to female population based controls. J Affect Disord 2003;75(1):77-82.

168. Wang H, Moser M, Schiltenwolf M, Buchner M. Circulating Cytokine Levels Compared to Pain in Patients with Fibromyalgia - A Prospective Longitudinal Study Over 6 Months. J Rheumatol 2008.

169. Amel Kashipaz MR, Swinden D, Todd I, Powell RJ. Normal production of inflammatory cytokines in chronic fatigue and fibromyalgia syndromes determined by intracellular cytokine staining in short-term cultured blood mononuclear cells. Clin Exp Immunol 2003;132(2):360-5.

170. Cuatrecasas G, Riudavets C, Guell MA, Nadal A. Growth hormone as concomitant treatment in severe fibromyalgia associated with low IGF-I serum levels. A pilot study. BMC Musculoskelet Disord 2007;8:119.

171. Tander B, Atmaca A, Aliyazicioglu Y, Canturk F. Serum ghrelin levels but not GH, IGF-I and IGFBP-3 levels are altered in patients with fibromyalgia syndrome. Joint Bone Spine 2007;74(5):477-81.

172. Altindag O, Gur A, Calgan N, Soran N, Celik H, Selek S. Paraoxonase and arylesterase activities in fibromyalgia. Redox Rep 2007;12(3):134-8.

173. Mease P. Fibromyalgia syndrome: review of clinical presentation, pathogenesis, outcome measures, and treatment. J Rheumatol Suppl 2005;75:6-21.

174. Lash AA, Ehrlich-Jones L, McCoy D. Fibromyalgia: evolving concepts and management in primary care settings. Medsurg Nurs 2003;12(3):145-59, 90; quiz 60.

175. Vaeroy H, Helle R, Forre O, Kass E, Terenius L. Elevated CSF levels of substance P and high incidence of Raynaud phenomenon in patients with fibromyalgia: new features for diagnosis. Pain 1988;32(1):21-6.

176. Leventhal LJ. Management of fibromyalgia. Ann Intern Med 1999;131(11):850-8.

177. Turk DC, Okifuji A, Sinclair JD, Starz TW. Differential responses by psychosocial subgroups of fibromyalgia syndrome patients to an interdisciplinary treatment. Arthritis Care Res 1998;11(5):397-404.

178. Thieme K, Rose U, Pinkpank T, Spies C, Turk DC, Flor H. Psychophysiological responses in patients with fibromyalgia syndrome. J Psychosom Res 2006;61(5):671-9.

179. Abeles M, Solitar BM, Pillinger MH, Abeles AM. Update on fibromyalgia therapy. Am J Med 2008;121(7):555-61.

180. Goldenberg DL, Simms RW, Geiger A, Komaroff AL. High frequency of fibromyalgia in patients with chronic fatigue seen in a primary care practice. Arthritis Rheum 1990;33(3):381-7.

181. Komaroff AL, Goldenberg D. The chronic fatigue syndrome: definition, current studies and lessons for fibromyalgia research. J Rheumatol Suppl 1989;19:23-7.

182. Whelton CL, Salit I, Moldofsky H. Sleep, Epstein-Barr virus infection, musculoskeletal pain, and depressive symptoms in chronic fatigue syndrome. J Rheumatol 1992;19(6):939-43.

183. Buchwald D. Fibromyalgia and chronic fatigue syndrome: similarities and differences. Rheum Dis Clin North Am 1996;22(2):219-43.

184. Buchwald D, Ashley RL, Pearlman T, Kith P, Komaroff AL. Viral serologies in patients with chronic fatigue and chronic fatigue syndrome. J Med Virol 1996;50(1):25-30.

185. Wallace HL, 2nd, Natelson B, Gause W, Hay J. Human herpesviruses in chronic fatigue syndrome. Clin Diagn Lab Immunol 1999;6(2):216-23.

186. Soto NE, Straus SE. Chronic Fatigue Syndrome and Herpesviruses: the Fading Evidence. Herpes 2000;7(2):46-50.

187. Depression. Mayo Foundation for Medical Education and Research, 2008. [Accessed Febryary 10, 2009, 2009, at

188. Roth T. The relationship between psychiatric diseases and insomnia. Int J Clin Pract Suppl 2001(116):3-8.

189. Lecrubier Y. Physical components of depression and psychomotor retardation. J Clin Psychiatry 2006;67 Suppl 6:23-6.

190. Fietta P, Fietta P, Manganelli P. Fibromyalgia and psychiatric disorders. Acta Biomed 2007;78(2):88-95.

191. Ahles TA, Yunus MB, Masi AT. Is chronic pain a variant of depressive disease? The case of primary fibromyalgia syndrome. Pain 1987;29(1):105-11.

192. Alfici S, Sigal M, Landau M. Primary fibromyalgia syndrome—a variant of depressive disorder? Psychother Psychosom 1989;51(3):156-61.

193. Goldenberg DL. Psychiatric and psychologic aspects of fibromyalgia syndrome. Rheum Dis Clin North Am 1989;15(1):105-14.

194. Ahles TA, Khan SA, Yunus MB, Spiegel DA, Masi AT. Psychiatric status of patients with primary fibromyalgia, patients with rheumatoid arthritis, and subjects without pain: a blind comparison of DSM-III diagnoses. Am J Psychiatry 1991;148(12):1721-6.

195. Sarzi-Puttini P, Buskila D, Carrabba M, Doria A, Atzeni F. Treatment strategy in fibromyalgia syndrome: where are we now? Semin Arthritis Rheum 2008;37(6):353-65.

196. Arnold LM. Duloxetine and other antidepressants in the treatment of patients with fibromyalgia. Pain Med 2007;8 Suppl 2:S63-74.

197. Dempsey J. Milnacipran for fibromyalgia. Issues Emerg Health Technol 2008(114):1-4.

198. Lawson K. Emerging pharmacological therapies for fibromyalgia. Curr Opin Investig Drugs 2006;7(7):631-6.

199. Lawrence RC, Felson DT, Helmick CG, Arnold LM, Choi H, Deyo RA, Gabriel S, Hirsch R, Hochberg MC, Hunder GG, Jordan JM, Katz JN, Kremers HM, Wolfe F. Estimates of the prevalence of arthritis and other rheumatic conditions in the United States. Part II. Arthritis Rheum 2008;58(1):26-35.

200. Helmick CG, Felson DT, Lawrence RC, Gabriel S, Hirsch R, Kwoh CK, Liang MH, Kremers HM, Mayes MD, Merkel PA, Pillemer SR, Reveille JD, Stone JH. Estimates of the prevalence of arthritis and other rheumatic conditions in the United States. Part I. Arthritis Rheum 2008;58(1):15-25.

201. Clauw DJ, Crofford LJ. Chronic widespread pain and fibromyalgia: what we know, and what we need to know. Best Pract Res Clin Rheumatol 2003;17(4):685-701.

202. Rudin NJ. Evaluation of treatments for myofascial pain syndrome and fibromyalgia. Curr Pain Headache Rep 2003;7(6):433-42.

203. Borg-Stein J. Treatment of fibromyalgia, myofascial pain, and related disorders. Phys Med Rehabil Clin N Am 2006;17(2):491-510, viii.

204. Gerwin RD. A review of myofascial pain and fibromyalgia--factors that promote their persistence. Acupunct Med 2005;23(3):121-34.

205. Borg-Stein J, Stein J. Trigger points and tender points: one and the same? Does injection treatment help? Rheum Dis Clin North Am 1996;22(2):305-22.

206. Harden RN, Bruehl SP, Gass S, Niemiec C, Barbick B. Signs and symptoms of the myofascial pain syndrome: a national survey of pain management providers. Clin J Pain 2000;16(1):64-72.

207. Bennett R. Myofascial pain syndromes and their evaluation. Best Pract Res Clin Rheumatol 2007;21(3):427-45.

208. Meyer HP. Myofascial pain syndrome and its suggested role in the pathogenesis and treatment of fibromyalgia syndrome. Curr Pain Headache Rep 2002;6(4):274-83.

209. Holland NW, Gonzalez EB. Soft tissue problems in older adults. Clin Geriatr Med 1998;14(3):601-11.

210. Gelberman RH, Hergenroeder PT, Hargens AR, Lundborg GN, Akeson WH. The carpal tunnel syndrome. A study of carpal canal pressures. J Bone Joint Surg Am 1981;63(3):380-3.

211. Lo SL, Raskin K, Lester H, Lester B. Carpal tunnel syndrome: a historical perspective. Hand Clin 2002;18(2):211-7, v.

212. McKenzie F, Storment J, Van Hook P, Armstrong TJ. A program for control of repetitive trauma disorders associated with hand tool operations in a telecommunications manufacturing facility. Am Ind Hyg Assoc J 1985;46(11):674-8.

213. Coke H, Seth-Smith D. Severe and active endocrine-metabolic type of arthritis. Rheumatism 1948;4(3):243.

214. Buchan JF. Acute gout and uric acid metabolism. Bras Med 1953;67(27-52):576-80.

215. Hoffman WS. Metabolism of uric acid and its relation to gout. J Am Med Assoc 1954;154(3):213-7.

216. Nugent CA, Tyler FH. The renal excretion of uric acid in patients with gout and in nongouty subjects. J Clin Invest 1959;38:1890-8.

217. Lawrence DJ, Meeker W, Branson R, Bronfort G, Cates JR, Haas M, Haneline M, Micozzi M, Updyke W, Mootz R, Triano JJ, Hawk C. Chiropractic management of low back pain and low back-related leg

complaints: a literature synthesis. J Manipulative Physiol Ther 2008;31(9):659-74.

218. Boyle KL, Demske JR. Management of a female with chronic sciatica and low back pain: a case report. Physiother Theory Pract 2009;25(1):44-54.

219. Yabuki S. Basic and update knowledge of intervertebral disc herniation: review. Fukushima J Med Sci 1999;45(2):63-75.

220. Sigal LH. Diagnosis of Lyme disease. Jama 1995;274(18):1427-8.

221. Bujak DI, Weinstein A, Dornbush RL. Clinical and neurocognitive features of the post Lyme syndrome. J Rheumatol 1996;23(8):1392-7.

222. Steere AC. Current understanding of Lyme disease. Hosp Pract [Off Ed] 1993;28(4):37-44.

223. Steere AC, Taylor E, McHugh GL, Logigian EL. The overdiagnosis of Lyme disease. Jama 1993;269(14):1812-6.

224. Bradley LA, McKendree-Smith NL, Alarcon GS, Cianfrini LR. Is fibromyalgia a neurologic disease? Curr Pain Headache Rep 2002;6(2):106-14.

225. Bennett R. The Fibromyalgia Impact Questionnaire [FIQ]: a review of its development, current version, operating characteristics and uses. Clin Exp Rheumatol 2005;23(5 Suppl 39):S154-62.

226. Zijlstra TR, Taal E, van de Laar MA, Rasker JJ. Validation of a Dutch translation of the fibromyalgia impact questionnaire. Rheumatology [Oxford] 2007;46(1):131-4.

227. Crofford LJ. Pain management in fibromyalgia. Curr Opin Rheumatol 2008;20(3):246-50.

228. Perrot S, Dickenson AH, Bennett RM. Fibromyalgia: harmonizing science with clinical practice considerations. Pain Pract 2008;8(3):177-89.

229. Harten P. [Fibromyalgia syndrome: new developments in pharmacotherapy]. Z Rheumatol 2008;67(1):75-82.

230. Ablin JN, Buskila D. Emerging therapies for fibromyalgia. Expert Opin Emerg Drugs 2008;13(1):53-62.

231. Owen RT. Pregabalin: its efficacy, safety and tolerability profile in fibromyalgia syndrome. Drugs Today [Barc] 2007;43(12):857-63.

232. [FDA approval for the antidepressive drug Cymbalta]. Krankenpfl J 2004;42(5-6):154.

233. Hussar DA. New drugs: milnacipran hydrochloride, fesoterodine fumarate, and silodosin. J Am Pharm Assoc [2003] 2009;49(2):347-50.

234. Mease PJ, Clauw DJ, Gendreau RM, Rao SG, Kranzler J, Chen W, Palmer RH. The efficacy and safety of milnacipran for treatment of fibromyalgia. a randomized, double-blind, placebo-controlled trial. J Rheumatol 2009;36(2):398-409.

235. Pae CU, Marks DC, Han C, Patkar AA, Masand PS. Duloxetine: an emerging evidence for fibromyalgia. Biomed Pharmacother 2009;63(1):69-71.

236. Duloxetine effective for fibromyalgia in some women. J Fam Pract 2006;55(5):382.

237. Leo RJ, Barkin RL. Antidepressant Use in Chronic Pain Management: Is There Evidence of a Role for Duloxetine? Prim Care Companion J Clin Psychiatry 2003;5(3):118-23.

238. Duloxetine (Cymbalta): a new SNRI for depression. Med Lett Drugs Ther 2004;46(1193):81-2.

239. Hunziker ME, Suehs BT, Bettinger TL, Crismon ML. Duloxetine hydrochloride: a new dual-acting medication for the treatment of major depressive disorder. Clin Ther 2005;27(8):1126-43.

240. Freedenfeld RN, Murray M, Fuchs PN, Kiser RS. Decreased pain and improved quality of life in fibromyalgia patients treated with olanzapine, an atypical neuroleptic. Pain Pract 2006;6(2):112-8.

241. Kiser RS, Cohen HM, Freedenfeld RN, Jewell C, Fuchs PN. Olanzapine for the treatment of fibromyalgia symptoms. J Pain Symptom Manage 2001;22(2):704-8.

242. Dooley DJ, Taylor CP, Donevan S, Feltner D. Ca2+ channel alpha2delta ligands: novel modulators of neurotransmission. Trends Pharmacol Sci 2007;28(2):75-82.

243. Arnold LM, Goldenberg DL, Stanford SB, Lalonde JK, Sandhu HS, Keck PE, Jr., Welge JA, Bishop F, Stanford KE, Hess EV, Hudson JI. Gabapentin in the treatment of fibromyalgia: a randomized, double-blind, placebo-controlled, multicenter trial. Arthritis Rheum 2007;56(4):1336-44.

244. Goldenberg DL. Pharmacological treatment of fibromyalgia and other chronic musculoskeletal pain. Best Pract Res Clin Rheumatol 2007;21(3):499-511.

245. Biasi G, Manca S, Manganelli S, Marcolongo R. Tramadol in the fibromyalgia syndrome: a controlled clinical trial versus placebo. Int J Clin Pharmacol Res 1998;18(1):13-9.

246. Foye WO, Lemke TL. Foye's principles of medicinal chemistry. 6th ed. Philadelphia: Lippincott Williams & Wilkins; 2008.

247. Vaeroy H, Abrahamsen A, Forre O, Kass E. Treatment of fibromyalgia (fibrositis syndrome): a parallel double blind trial with carisoprodol, paracetamol and caffeine (Somadril comp) versus placebo. Clin Rheumatol 1989;8(2):245-50.

248. Abruzzi WA. A Controlled Evaluation of Chlorphenesin Carbamate in Painful Musculoskeletal Syndromes. Clin Med (Northfield Il) 1964;71:329-48.

249. Casale R, Tugnoli V. Botulinum toxin for pain. Drugs R D 2008;9(1):11-27.

250. Ferreira JJ, Couto M, Costa J, Coelho M, Rosa MM, Sampaio C. [Botulinum toxin for the treatment of pain syndromes]. Acta Reumatol Port 2006;31(1):49-62.

251. Staud R. Are tender point injections beneficial: the role of tonic nociception in fibromyalgia. Curr Pharm Des 2006;12(1):23-7.

252. Smith HS, Audette J, Royal MA. Botulinum toxin in pain management of soft tissue syndromes. Clin J Pain 2002;18(6 Suppl):S147-54.

253. Sheean G. Botulinum toxin for the treatment of musculoskeletal pain and spasm. Curr Pain Headache Rep 2002;6(6):460-9.

254. Benecke R, Dressler D, Kunesch E, Probst T. [Use of botulinum toxin the the treatment of muscle pain]. Schmerz 2003;17(6):450-8.

255. Paulson GW, Gill W. Botulinum toxin is unsatisfactory therapy for fibromyalgia. Mov Disord 1996;11(4):459.

256. Carette S, McCain GA, Bell DA, Fam AG. Evaluation of amitriptyline in primary fibrositis. A double-blind, placebo-controlled study. Arthritis Rheum 1986;29(5):655-9.

257. Goldenberg DL. A review of the role of tricyclic medications in the treatment of fibromyalgia syndrome. J Rheumatol Suppl 1989;19:137-9.

258. Goldenberg DL, Felson DT, Dinerman H. A randomized, controlled trial of amitriptyline and naproxen in the treatment of patients with fibromyalgia. Arthritis Rheum 1986;29(11):1371-7.

259. Scudds RA, McCain GA, Rollman GB, Harth M. Improvements in pain responsiveness in patients with fibrositis after successful treatment with amitriptyline. J Rheumatol Suppl 1989;19:98-103.

260. Carette S, Bell MJ, Reynolds WJ, Haraoui B, McCain GA, Bykerk VP, Edworthy SM, Baron M, Koehler BE, Fam AG, et al. Comparison of amitriptyline, cyclobenzaprine, and placebo in the treatment of fibromyalgia. A randomized, double-blind clinical trial. Arthritis Rheum 1994;37(1):32-40.

261. Share NN. Cyclobenzaprine: studies on its site of muscle relaxant action in the cat. Neuropharmacology 1980;19(8):757-64.

262. Share NN, McFarlane CS. Cyclobenzaprine: novel centrally acting skeletal muscle relaxant. Neuropharmacology 1975;14(9):675-84.

263. Bennett RM, Gatter RA, Campbell SM, Andrews RP, Clark SR, Scarola JA. A comparison of cyclobenzaprine and placebo in the management of fibrositis. A double-blind controlled study. Arthritis Rheum 1988;31(12):1535-42.

264. Romano TJ. Fibromyalgia in children; diagnosis and treatment. W V Med J 1991;87(3):112-4.

265. Arnold LM, Hess EV, Hudson JI, Welge JA, Berno SE, Keck PE, Jr. A randomized, placebo-controlled, double-blind, flexible-dose study of fluoxetine in the treatment of women with fibromyalgia. Am J Med 2002;112(3):191-7.

266. Nerhood RC. Fluoxetine and pregnancy a safe mix? Postgrad Med 1998;104(5):37-8.

267. Finestone DH, Ober SK. Fluoxetine and fibromyalgia. Jama 1990;264(22):2869-70.

268. Geller SA. Treatment of fibrositis with fluoxetine hydrochloride (Prozac). Am J Med 1989;87(5):594-5.

269. Patkar AA, Masand PS, Krulewicz S, Mannelli P, Peindl K, Beebe KL, Jiang W. A randomized, controlled, trial of controlled release paroxetine in fibromyalgia. Am J Med 2007;120(5):448-54.

270. Bazzichi L, Giannaccini G, Betti L, Mascia G, Fabbrini L, Italiani P, De Feo F, Giuliano T, Giacomelli C, Rossi A, Lucacchini A, Bombardieri S. Alteration of serotonin transporter density and activity in fibromyalgia. Arthritis Res Ther 2006;8(4):R99.

271. Hathcock JN, Shao A, Vieth R, Heaney R. Risk assessment for vitamin D. Am J Clin Nutr 2007;85(1):6-18.

272. Hathcock J. Tolerable upper intake level of vitamin D. Am J Clin Nutr 2001;74(6):864-5; author reply 6-7.

273. Shinchuk LM, Holick MF. Vitamin d and rehabilitation: improving functional outcomes. Nutr Clin Pract 2007;22(3):297-304.

274. Faiz S, Panunti B, Andrews S. The epidemic of vitamin D deficiency. J La State Med Soc 2007;159(1):17-20; quiz , 55.

275. Erkal MZ, Wilde J, Bilgin Y, Akinci A, Demir E, Bodeker RH, Mann M, Bretzel RG, Stracke H, Holick MF. High prevalence of vitamin D deficiency, secondary hyperparathyroidism and generalized bone pain in Turkish immigrants in Germany: identification of risk factors. Osteoporos Int 2006;17(8):1133-40.

276. Block SR. Vitamin D deficiency is not associated with nonspecific musculoskeletal pain syndromes including fibromyalgia. Mayo Clin Proc 2004;79(12):1585-6; author reply 6-7.

277. Holick MF. Vitamin D: importance in the prevention of cancers, type 1 diabetes, heart disease, and osteoporosis. Am J Clin Nutr 2004;79(3):362-71.

278. Al-Allaf AW, Mole PA, Paterson CR, Pullar T. Bone health in patients with fibromyalgia. Rheumatology (Oxford) 2003;42(10):1202-6.

279. Warner AE, Arnspiger SA. Diffuse musculoskeletal pain is not associated with low vitamin D levels or improved by treatment with vitamin D. J Clin Rheumatol 2008;14(1):12-6.

280. Gaby AR. Intravenous nutrient therapy: the "Myers' cocktail". Altern Med Rev 2002;7(5):389-403.

281. Massey PB. Reduction of fibromyalgia symptoms through intravenous nutrient therapy: results of a pilot clinical trial. Altern Ther Health Med 2007;13(3):32-4.

282. Lonsdale D, Shamberger RJ, Stahl JP, Evans R. Evaluation of the biochemical effects of administration of intravenous nutrients using erythrocyte ATP/ADP ratios. Altern Med Rev 1999;4(1):37-44.

283. Citera G, Arias MA, Maldonado-Cocco JA, Lazaro MA, Rosemffet MG, Brusco LI, Scheines EJ, Cardinalli DP. The effect of melatonin in patients with fibromyalgia: a pilot study. Clin Rheumatol 2000;19(1):9-13.

284. Press J, Phillip M, Neumann L, Barak R, Segev Y, Abu-Shakra M, Buskila D. Normal melatonin levels in patients with fibromyalgia syndrome. J Rheumatol 1998;25(3):551-5.

285. Korszun A, Sackett-Lundeen L, Papadopoulos E, Brucksch C, Masterson L, Engelberg NC, Haus E, Demitrack MA, Crofford L. Melatonin levels in women with fibromyalgia and chronic fatigue syndrome. J Rheumatol 1999;26(12):2675-80.

286. Sadreddini S, Molaeefard M, Noshad H, Ardalan M, Asadi A. Efficacy of Raloxifen in treatment of fibromyalgia in menopausal women. Eur J Intern Med 2008;19(5):350-5.

287. Toda K, Tobimatsu Y. Efficacy of neurotropin in fibromyalgia: a case report. Pain Med 2008;9(4):460-3.

288. Toda K, Kimura H. Efficacy of neurotropin in chronic fatigue syndrome: a case report. Hiroshima J Med Sci 2006;55(1):35-7.

289. Wolfe F, Anderson J, Harkness D, Bennett RM, Caro XJ, Goldenberg DL, Russell IJ, Yunus MB. Health status and disease severity in fibromyalgia: results of a six-center longitudinal study. Arthritis Rheum 1997;40(9):1571-9.

290. Weaver M, Schnoll S. Abuse liability in opioid therapy for pain treatment in patients with an addiction history. Clin J Pain 2002;18(4 Suppl):S61-9.

291. Aronoff GM. Opioids in chronic pain management: is there a significant risk of addiction? Curr Rev Pain 2000;4(2):112-21.

292. Miotto K, Compton P, Ling W, Conolly M. Diagnosing addictive disease in chronic pain patients. Psychosomatics 1996;37(3):223-35.

293. Jung B, Reidenberg MM. The risk of action by the Drug Enforcement Administration against physicians prescribing opioids for pain. Pain Med 2006;7(4):353-7.

294. Sorensen J, Bengtsson A, Ahlner J, Henriksson KG, Ekselius L, Bengtsson M. Fibromyalgia--are there different mechanisms in the processing of pain? A double blind crossover comparison of analgesic drugs. J Rheumatol 1997;24(8):1615-21.

295. Graven-Nielsen T, Aspegren Kendall S, Henriksson KG, Bengtsson M, Sorensen J, Johnson A, Gerdle B, Arendt-Nielsen L. Ketamine reduces muscle pain, temporal summation, and referred pain in fibromyalgia patients. Pain 2000;85(3):483-91.

296. Koppert W, Zeck S, Sittl R, Likar R, Knoll R, Schmelz M. Low-dose lidocaine suppresses experimentally induced hyperalgesia in humans. Anesthesiology 1998;89(6):1345-53.

297. Oye I, Rabben T, Fagerlund TH. [Analgesic effect of ketamine in a patient with neuropathic pain]. Tidsskr Nor Laegeforen 1996;116(26):3130-1.

298. Scherer FM. The pharmaceutical industry—prices and progress. N Engl J Med 2004;351(9):927-32.

299. Reichert JM. New biopharmaceuticals in the USA: trends in development and marketing approvals 1995-1999. Trends Biotechnol 2000;18(9):364-9.

300. Epstein JH. Experimental models for primary melanoma. Photodermatol Photoimmunol Photomed 1992;9(3):91-8.

301. Avon SL, Wood RE. Porcine skin as an in-vivo model for ageing of human bite marks. J Forensic Odontostomatol 2005;23(2):30-9.

302. Cummings BJ, Head E, Ruehl W, Milgram NW, Cotman CW. The canine as an animal model of human aging and dementia. Neurobiol Aging 1996;17(2):259-68.

303. Genao A, Seth K, Schmidt U, Carles M, Gwathmey JK. Dilated cardiomyopathy in turkeys: an animal model for the study of human heart failure. Lab Anim Sci 1996;46(4):399-404.

304. Han Lee ED, Kemball CC, Wang J, Dong Y, Stapler DC, Jr., Hamby KM, Gangappa S, Newell KA, Pearson TC, Lukacher AE, Larsen CP. A mouse model for polyomavirus-associated nephropathy of kidney transplants. Am J Transplant 2006;6(5 Pt 1):913-22.

305. Tsuji Y, Ariyoshi A, Sakamoto K. An experimental model for unilateral ischaemic acute renal failure in dog. Int Urol Nephrol 1993;25(1):83-8.

306. Miyasaka K, Funakoshi A. Is the OLETF rat a good model of central sensitization? J Pharmacol Sci 2007;105(4):373.

307. Felix FH, Fontenele JB. The OLETF rat as a model of central sensitization: possible relevance to the study of fibromyalgia and related diseases. J Pharmacol Sci 2007;105(4):372.

308. Russell IJ. Advances in fibromyalgia: possible role for central neurochemicals. Am J Med Sci 1998;315(6):377-84.

309. Nishiyori M, Ueda H. Prolonged gabapentin analgesia in an experimental mouse model of fibromyalgia. Mol Pain 2008;4:52.

310. Rosner F. Is animal experimentation being threatened by animal rights groups? Jama 1985;254(14):1942-3.

311. Dawson J. Animal experiments: conference report. Br Med J (Clin Res Ed) 1986;292(6536):1654-5.

312. Brainard J. Animal-rights groups fight colleges over access to research records. Chron High Educ 2006;52(30):A29.

313. Sechzer JA. Historical issues concerning animal experimentation in the United States. Soc Sci Med 1981;15F:13-7.

314. Bulger RE. Use of animals in experimental research: a scientist's perspective. Anat Rec 1987;219(3):215-20.

315. Wigley R. When is a placebo effect not an effect? Clin Med 2007;7(5):450-2.

316. Colloca L, Benedetti F, Porro CA. Experimental designs and brain mapping approaches for studying the placebo analgesic effect. Eur J Appl Physiol 2008;102(4):371-80.

317. Lidstone SC, Stoessl AJ. Understanding the placebo effect: contributions from neuroimaging. Mol Imaging Biol 2007;9(4):176-85.

318. Crum AJ, Langer EJ. Mind-set matters: exercise and the placebo effect. Psychol Sci 2007;18(2):165-71.

319. Reichert S, Simon T, Halm EA. Physicians' attitudes about prescribing and knowledge of the costs of common medications. Arch Intern Med 2000;160(18):2799-803.

320. Gusi N, Tomas-Carus P. Cost-utility of an 8-month aquatic training for women with fibromyalgia: a randomized controlled trial. Arthritis Res Ther 2008;10(1):R24.

321. Gusi N, Tomas-Carus P, Hakkinen A, Hakkinen K, Ortega-Alonso A. Exercise in waist-high warm water decreases pain and improves health-related quality of life and strength in the lower extremities in women with fibromyalgia. Arthritis Rheum 2006;55(1):66-73.

322. Mannerkorpi K, Ahlmen M, Ekdahl C. Six- and 24-month follow-up of pool exercise therapy and education for patients with fibromyalgia. Scand J Rheumatol 2002;31(5):306-10.

323. Donmez A, Karagulle MZ, Tercan N, Dinler M, Issever H, Karagulle M, Turan M. SPA therapy in fibromyalgia: a randomised controlled clinic study. Rheumatol Int 2005;26(2):168-72.

324. Altan L, Bingol U, Aykac M, Koc Z, Yurtkuran M. Investigation of the effects of pool-based exercise on fibromyalgia syndrome. Rheumatol Int 2004;24(5):272-7.

325. Grossman P, Tiefenthaler-Gilmer U, Raysz A, Kesper U. Mindfulness training as an intervention for fibromyalgia: evidence of postintervention and 3-year follow-up benefits in well-being. Psychother Psychosom 2007;76(4):226-33.

326. Wahbeh H, Elsas SM, Oken BS. Mind-body interventions: applications in neurology. Neurology 2008;70(24):2321-8.

327. da Silva GD, Lorenzi-Filho G, Lage LV. Effects of yoga and the addition of Tui Na in patients with fibromyalgia. J Altern Complement Med 2007;13(10):1107-13.

328. Haak T, Scott B. The effect of Qigong on Fibromyalgia (FMS): A controlled randomized study. Disabil Rehabil 2007:1-9.

329. Taggart HM, Arslanian CL, Bae S, Singh K. Effects of T'ai Chi exercise on fibromyalgia symptoms and health-related quality of life. Orthop Nurs 2003;22(5):353-60.

330. Langhorst J, Hauser W, Irnich D, Speeck N, Felde E, Winkelmann A, Lucius H, Michalsen A, Musial F. [Alternative and complementary therapies in fibromyalgia syndrome.]. Schmerz 2008;22(3):324-33.

331. Dobkin PL, Da Costa D, Abrahamowicz M, Dritsa M, Du Berger R, Fitzcharles MA, Lowensteyn I. Adherence during an individualized home based 12-week exercise program in women with fibromyalgia. J Rheumatol 2006;33(2):333-41.

332. Dobkin PL, Abrahamowicz M, Fitzcharles MA, Dritsa M, da Costa D. Maintenance of exercise in women with fibromyalgia. Arthritis Rheum 2005;53(5):724-31.

333. Mannerkorpi K, Henriksson C. Non-pharmacological treatment of chronic widespread musculoskeletal pain. Best Pract Res Clin Rheumatol 2007;21(3):513-34.

334. Burckhardt CS. Educating patients: self-management approaches. Disabil Rehabil 2005;27(12):703-9.

335. Gowans SE, deHueck A. Effectiveness of exercise in management of fibromyalgia. Curr Opin Rheumatol 2004;16(2):138-42.

336. Offenbacher M, Stucki G. Physical therapy in the treatment of fibromyalgia. Scand J Rheumatol Suppl 2000;113:78-85.

337. Shaver JL, Wilbur J, Robinson FP, Wang E, Buntin MS. Women's health issues with fibromyalgia syndrome. J Womens Health (Larchmt) 2006;15(9):1035-45.

338. Glass JM, Lyden AK, Petzke F, Stein P, Whalen G, Ambrose K, Chrousos G, Clauw DJ. The effect of brief exercise cessation on pain, fatigue, and mood symptom development in healthy, fit individuals. J Psychosom Res 2004;57(4):391-8.

339. Ambrose K, Lyden AK, Clauw DJ. Applying exercise to the management of fibromyalgia. Curr Pain Headache Rep 2003;7(5):348-54.

340. Mannerkorpi K. Exercise in fibromyalgia. Curr Opin Rheumatol 2005;17(2):190-4.

341. Evans WJ. Protein nutrition, exercise and aging. J Am Coll Nutr 2004;23(6 Suppl):601S-9S.

342. Rhodes EC, Martin AD, Taunton JE, Donnelly M, Warren J, Elliot J. Effects of one year of resistance training on the relation between muscular strength and bone density in elderly women. Br J Sports Med 2000;34(1):18-22.

343. Cussler EC, Lohman TG, Going SB, Houtkooper LB, Metcalfe LL, Flint-Wagner HG, Harris RB, Teixeira PJ. Weight lifted in strength training

predicts bone change in postmenopausal women. Med Sci Sports Exerc 2003;35(1):10-7.

344. Going S, Lohman T, Houtkooper L, Metcalfe L, Flint-Wagner H, Blew R, Stanford V, Cussler E, Martin J, Teixeira P, Harris M, Milliken L, Figueroa-Galvez A, Weber J. Effects of exercise on bone mineral density in calcium-replete postmenopausal women with and without hormone replacement therapy. Osteoporos Int 2003;14(8):637-43.

345. Maddalozzo GF, Snow CM. High intensity resistance training: effects on bone in older men and women. Calcif Tissue Int 2000;66(6):399-404.

346. Hakkinen A, Sokka T, Kotaniemi A, Hannonen P. A randomized two-year study of the effects of dynamic strength training on muscle strength, disease activity, functional capacity, and bone mineral density in early rheumatoid arthritis. Arthritis Rheum 2001;44(3):515-22.

347. Deschenes MR, Kraemer WJ. Performance and physiologic adaptations to resistance training. Am J Phys Med Rehabil 2002;81(11 Suppl):S3-16.

348. Hobson K. The stronger sex. Women who lift weights get healthier, better bodies--not, new research shows, bulkier ones. US News World Rep 2002;132(16):52-3.

349. Gur A. Physical therapy modalities in management of fibromyalgia. Curr Pharm Des 2006;12(1):29-35.

350. Morris CR, Bowen L, Morris AJ. Integrative therapy for fibromyalgia: possible strategies for an individualized treatment program. South Med J 2005;98(2):177-84.

351. Assefi NP, Sherman KJ, Jacobsen C, Goldberg J, Smith WR, Buchwald D. A randomized clinical trial of acupuncture compared with sham acupuncture in fibromyalgia. Ann Intern Med 2005;143(1):10-9.

352. Martin DP, Sletten CD, Williams BA, Berger IH. Improvement in fibromyalgia symptoms with acupuncture: results of a randomized controlled trial. Mayo Clin Proc 2006;81(6):749-57.

353. Lundeberg T, Lund I. Did 'The Princess on the Pea' suffer from fibromyalgia syndrome? The influence on sleep and the effects of acupuncture. Acupunct Med 2007;25(4):184-97.

354. Harris RE, Tian X, Williams DA, Tian TX, Cupps TR, Petzke F, Groner KH, Biswas P, Gracely RH, Clauw DJ. Treatment of fibromyalgia with formula acupuncture: investigation of needle placement, needle stimulation, and treatment frequency. J Altern Complement Med 2005;11(4):663-71.

355. Cabyoglu MT, Ergene N, Tan U. The mechanism of acupuncture and clinical applications. Int J Neurosci 2006;116(2):115-25.

356. Brattberg G. Connective tissue massage in the treatment of fibromyalgia. Eur J Pain 1999;3(3):235-44.

357. Barbour C. Use of complementary and alternative treatments by individuals with fibromyalgia syndrome. J Am Acad Nurse Pract 2000;12(8):311-6.

358. Maurizio SJ, Rogers JL. Recognizing and treating fibromyalgia. Nurse Pract 1997;22(12):18-26, 8, 31; quiz 2-3.

359. Galloway J. Maintaining serenity in chronic illness. N Y State J Med 1990;90(7):366-7.

360. van Uden-Kraan CF, Drossaert CH, Taal E, Shaw BR, Seydel ER, van de Laar MA. Empowering processes and outcomes of participation in online support groups for patients with breast cancer, arthritis, or fibromyalgia. Qual Health Res 2008;18(3):405-17.

361. Barker KK. Electronic support groups, patient-consumers, and medicalization: the case of contested illness. J Health Soc Behav 2008;49(1):20-36.

362. Goossens ME, Rutten-van Molken MP, Leidl RM, Bos SG, Vlaeyen JW, Teeken-Gruben NJ. Cognitive-educational treatment of fibromyalgia: a randomized clinical trial. II. Economic evaluation. J Rheumatol 1996;23(7):1246-54.

363. Vlaeyen JW, Teeken-Gruben NJ, Goossens ME, Rutten-van Molken MP, Pelt RA, van Eek H, Heuts PH. Cognitive-educational treatment of fibromyalgia: a randomized clinical trial. I. Clinical effects. J Rheumatol 1996;23(7):1237-45.

364. Ottonello M. Cognitive-behavioral interventions in rheumatic diseases. G Ital Med Lav Ergon 2007;29(1 Suppl A):A19-23.

365. Staud R. Treatment of fibromyalgia and its symptoms. Expert Opin Pharmacother 2007;8(11):1629-42.

366. Werner A, Malterud K. It is hard work behaving as a credible patient: encounters between women with chronic pain and their doctors. Soc Sci Med 2003;57(8):1409-19.

367. Merskey H. Social influences on the concept of fibromyalgia. CNS Spectr 2008;13(3 Suppl 5):18-21.

368. McDermott BE, Feldman MD. Malingering in the medical setting. Psychiatr Clin North Am 2007;30(4):645-62.

369. Segal JZ. Illness as argumentation: a prolegomenon to the rhetorical study of contestable complaints. Health (London) 2007;11(2):227-44.

370. Mittenberg W, Patton C, Canyock EM, Condit DC. Base rates of malingering and symptom exaggeration. J Clin Exp Neuropsychol 2002;24(8):1094-102.

371. Rothschild BM. Fibromyalgia: can one distinguish it from simulation? J Rheumatol 2001;28(12):2762-3.

372. Gervais RO, Russell AS, Green P, Allen LM, 3rd, Ferrari R, Pieschl SD. Effort testing in patients with fibromyalgia and disability incentives. J Rheumatol 2001;28(8):1892-9.

373. Wolfe F. Sayin' "stand and deliver, for you are a bold deceiver": faking fibromyalgia. J Rheumatol 2000;27(11):2534-5.

374. Rau CL, Russell IJ. Is fibromyalgia a distinct clinical syndrome? Curr Rev Pain 2000;4(4):287-94.

375. Keefe FJ, Caldwell DS. Cognitive behavioral control of arthritis pain. Med Clin North Am 1997;81(1):277-90.

376. Cronan TA, Serber ER, Walen HR, Jaffe M. The influence of age on fibromyalgia symptoms. J Aging Health 2002;14(3):370-84.

377. Romano TJ. Clinical experiences with post-traumatic fibromyalgia syndrome. W V Med J 1990;86(5):198-202.

378. Romano TJ. Fibromyalgia and the law. J Rheumatol 2001;28(3):674; author reply 5-8.

379. Hadler NM, Ehrlich GE. Fibromyalgia and the conundrum of disability determination. J Occup Environ Med 2003;45(10):1030-3.

380. Johnson M, Paananen ML, Rahinantti P, Hannonen P. Depressed fibromyalgia patients are equipped with an emphatic competence dependent self-esteem. Clin Rheumatol 1997;16(6):578-84.

381. Ventegodt S, Gringols M, Merrick J. Clinical holistic medicine: whiplash, fibromyalgia, and chronic fatigue. ScientificWorldJournal 2005;5:340-54.

382. Schur EA, Afari N, Furberg H, Olarte M, Goldberg J, Sullivan PF, Buchwald D. Feeling bad in more ways than one: comorbidity patterns of medically unexplained and psychiatric conditions. J Gen Intern Med 2007;22(6):818-21.

383. Buskila D, Cohen H. Comorbidity of fibromyalgia and psychiatric disorders. Curr Pain Headache Rep 2007;11(5):333-8.

384. Palomino RA, Nicassio PM, Greenberg MA, Medina EP, Jr. Helplessness and loss as mediators between pain and depressive symptoms in fibromyalgia. Pain 2007;129(1-2):185-94.

385. Cook DB, Stegner AJ, McLoughlin MJ. Imaging pain of fibromyalgia. Curr Pain Headache Rep 2007;11(3):190-200.

386. Nelson PJ, Tucker S. Developing an intervention to alter catastrophizing in persons with fibromyalgia. Orthop Nurs 2006;25(3):205-14.

387. Wolfe F, Anderson J, Harkness D, Bennett RM, Caro XJ, Goldenberg DL, Russell IJ, Yunus MB. Work and disability status of persons with fibromyalgia. J Rheumatol 1997;24(6):1171-8.

388. Munce SE, Stewart DE. Gender differences in depression and chronic pain conditions in a national epidemiologic survey. Psychosomatics 2007;48(5):394-9.

389. Munce SE, Stansfeld SA, Blackmore ER, Stewart DE. The role of depression and chronic pain conditions in absenteeism: results from a national epidemiologic survey. J Occup Environ Med 2007;49(11):1206-11.

390. Stenager EN, Svendsen MA, Stenager E. [Disability retirement pension for patients with syndrome diagnoses. A registry study on the basis of data from the Social Appeal Board]. Ugeskr Laeger 2003;165(5):469-74.

391. Al-Allaf AW. Work disability and health system utilization in patients with fibromyalgia syndrome. J Clin Rheumatol 2007;13(4):199-201.

392. Wolfe F, Potter J. Fibromyalgia and work disability: Is Fibromyalgia a disabling disorder? Rheum Dis Clin North Am 1996;22(2):369-91.

393. United States Federal Government. Americans with Disabilities Act of 1990. Public Law No. 101-336. US Statut Large 1990;104:327-78.

394. Beger CS. The importance of subjective claims management. Benefits Q 1997;13(4):41-5.

395. Coetzer P, Lockyer I, Schorn D, Boshoff L. Assessing impairment and disability for syndromes presenting with chronic fatigue. J Insur Med 2001;33(2):170-82.

396. Yunus MB, Masi AT. Juvenile primary fibromyalgia syndrome. A clinical study of thirty-three patients and matched normal controls. Arthritis Rheum 1985;28(2):138-45.

397. Calabro JJ. Fibromyalgia (fibrositis) in children. Am J Med 1986;81(3A):57-9.

398. Breau LM, McGrath PJ, Ju LH. Review of juvenile primary fibromyalgia and chronic fatigue syndrome. J Dev Behav Pediatr 1999;20(4):278-88.

399. Walco GA, Ilowite NT. Cognitive-behavioral intervention for juvenile primary fibromyalgia syndrome. J Rheumatol 1992;19(10):1617-9.

400. Schanberg LE, Keefe FJ, Lefebvre JC, Kredich DW, Gil KM. Pain coping strategies in children with juvenile primary fibromyalgia syndrome: correlation with pain, physical function, and psychological distress. Arthritis Care Res 1996;9(2):89-96.

401. Yunus MB, Arslan S, Aldag JC. Relationship between body mass index and fibromyalgia features. Scand J Rheumatol 2002;31(1):27-31.

402. Ogden CL, Yanovski SZ, Carroll MD, Flegal KM. The epidemiology of obesity. Gastroenterology 2007;132(6):2087-102.

403. Quinzi DR. Obesity in children. Adv Nurse Pract 1999;7(3):46-50.

404. de Sa Pinto AL, de Barros Holanda PM, Radu AS, Villares SM, Lima FR. Musculoskeletal findings in obese children. J Paediatr Child Health 2006;42(6):341-4.

405. Hooper MM, Stellato TA, Hallowell PT, Seitz BA, Moskowitz RW. Musculoskeletal findings in obese subjects before and after weight loss following bariatric surgery. Int J Obes (Lond) 2007;31(1):114-20.

406. Shapiro JR, Anderson DA, Danoff-Burg S. A pilot study of the effects of behavioral weight loss treatment on fibromyalgia symptoms. J Psychosom Res 2005;59(5):275-82.

407. Haugen M, Kjeldsen-Kragh J, Nordvag BY, Forre O. Diet and disease symptoms in rheumatic diseases--results of a questionnaire based survey. Clin Rheumatol 1991;10(4):401-7.

408. Tayag-Kier CE, Keenan GF, Scalzi LV, Schultz B, Elliott J, Zhao RH, Arens R. Sleep and periodic limb movement in sleep in juvenile fibromyalgia. Pediatrics 2000;106(5):E70.

409. Kashikar-Zuck S, Lynch AM, Graham TB, Swain NF, Mullen SM, Noll RB. Social functioning and peer relationships of adolescents with juvenile fibromyalgia syndrome. Arthritis Rheum 2007;57(3):474-80.

410. Reid GJ, McGrath PJ, Lang BA. Parent-child interactions among children with juvenile fibromyalgia, arthritis, and healthy controls. Pain 2005;113(1-2):201-10.

411. Schanberg LE, Keefe FJ, Lefebvre JC, Kredich DW, Gil KM. Social context of pain in children with Juvenile Primary Fibromyalgia Syndrome: parental pain history and family environment. Clin J Pain 1998;14(2):107-15.

412. Brown GT, Delisle R, Gagnon N, Sauve AE. Juvenile fibromyalgia syndrome: proposed management using a cognitive-behavioral approach. Phys Occup Ther Pediatr 2001;21(1):19-36.

413. Saccomani L, Vigliarolo MA, Sbolgi P, Ruffa G, Doria Lamba L. [Juvenile fibromyalgia syndrome: 2 clinical cases]. Pediatr Med Chir 1993;15(1):99-101.

414. Coster L, Kendall S, Gerdle B, Henriksson C, Henriksson KG, Bengtsson A. Chronic widespread musculoskeletal pain - a comparison of those who meet criteria for fibromyalgia and those who do not. Eur J Pain 2008;12(5):600-10.

Notes